HEALTH ASSESSMENT

& Physical Examination

Student Lab Manual

Mary Ellen Zator Estes, RN, MSN, CCRN
Assistant Professor
School of Nursing
Marymount University
Arlington, Virginia
and
Former Critical Care Nursing Education Coordinator
The George Washington University Medical Center
Washington, D.C.

Prepared by
Kathleen Peck Schaefer, RNC, MSN, MEd
Clinical Instructor, Adjunct Faculty
School of Nursing
Marymount University
Arlington, Virginia
and
Nursing Staff
Fairfax Hospital
Falls Church, Virginia

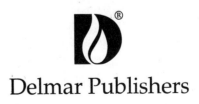

Delmar Publishers

I(T)P® an International Thomson Publishing company

Albany • Bonn • Boston • Cincinnati • Detroit • London • Madrid
Melbourne • Mexico City • New York • Pacific Grove • Paris • San Francisco
Singapore • Tokyo • Toronto • Washington

Cover Design: Brucie Rosch
The cover photograph illustrates the assessment for Tinel's sign, a test for the carpal tunnel syndrome.

Delmar Staff
Publisher: William Brottmiller
Acquisitions Editor: Cathy L. Esperti
Developmental Editor: Elisabeth F. Williams
Project Editor: Patricia Gillivan
Production Coordinator: Barbara A. Bullock
Art and Design Coordinator: Timothy J. Conners

COPYRIGHT © 1998
Delmar is a division of Thomson Learning. The Thomson Learning logo is a registered trademark used herein under license.

Printed in the United States of America
3 4 5 6 7 8 9 10 XXX 04 03 02 01 00

For more information, contact Delmar, 3 Columbia Circle, PO Box 15015, Albany, NY 12212-0515; or find us on the World Wide Web at http://www.delmar.com

International Division List

Japan:
Thomson Learning
Palaceside Building 5F
1-1-1 Hitotsubashi, Chiyoda-ku
Tokyo 100 0003 Japan
Tel: 813 5218 6544
Fax: 813 5218 6551

Australia/New Zealand:
Nelson/Thomson Learning
102 Dodds Street
South Melbourne, Victoria 3205
Australia
Tel: 61 39 685 4111
Fax: 61 39 685 4199

UK/Europe/Middle East:
Thomson Learning
Berkshire House
168-173 High Holborn
London
WC1V 7AA United Kingdom
Tel: 44 171 497 1422
Fax: 44 171 497 1426

Latin America:
Thomson Learning
Seneca, 53
Colonia Polanco
11560 Mexico D.F. Mexico
Tel: 525-281-2906
Fax: 525-281-2656

Canada:
Nelson/Thomson Learning
1120 Birchmount Road
Scarborough, Ontario
Canada M1K 5G4
Tel: 416-752-9100
Fax: 416-752-8102

Asia:
Thomson Learning
60 Albert Street, #15-01
Albert Complex
Singapore 189969
Tel: 65 336 6411
Fax: 65 336 7411

Library of Congress Card Number: 97-13500
CIP
ISBN: 0-7668-0911-0

Contents

Preface

This lab manual is designed to accompany *Health Assessment & Physical Examination* by Mary Ellen Zator Estes, RN, MSN, CCRN. Each of the 24 chapters in this lab manual is developed to facilitate student learning of health assessment skills in a varied format. By using this lab manual at home and in the laboratory setting, nursing students will work with important concepts and begin to apply them to real-life situations.

As a clinical/lab instructor, I have developed guides and quizzes to help students grasp the concepts and procedures in clinical nursing. I have found that injecting a little humor in certain instances facilitates this learning process. The nursing laboratory can and should be a center of dynamic instruction and learning. Enthusiastic and creative instructors, provided with resources that include well-developed laboratory guides, help students acquire the skills needed for competent and compassionate nursing care. As the patient population becomes increasingly diverse and ill, the nurse's health assessment skills become more essential, and the use of a lab manual to enhance student learning gains importance. This lab manual provides a guide for that learning.

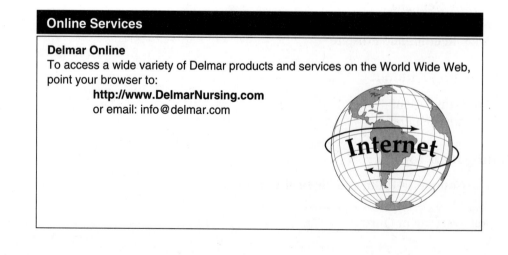

Online Services

Delmar Online
To access a wide variety of Delmar products and services on the World Wide Web, point your browser to:
        http://www.DelmarNursing.com
        or email: info@delmar.com

Lab Practice for The Nursing Process

Learning Objectives

1. Identify the phases of the nursing process.
2. Determine the information sources for the assessment process.
3. Formulate nursing diagnoses.
4. Compare nursing care plans and critical pathways.

Reading Assignment

Prior to beginning this lab assignment, please read Chapter 1, "The Nursing Process," in *Health Assessment & Physical Examination* by Mary Ellen Zator Estes, pages 3–16.

Key Terms

Please define the following terms:

Actual Nursing Diagnosis _____

_____

Assessment _____

_____

Clustering _____

_____

Collaborative Intervention _____

_____

Collaborative Problem _____

_____

Critical Pathway _____

_____

Defining Characteristics _____

_____

Descriptor or Qualifier _____

_____

Evaluation _____

_____

Functional Health Patterns _____

_____

Human Response Patterns _____

_____

Implementation _____

_____

Independent Nursing Interventions _____

_____

Intervention _____

_____

Long-Term Outcome _____

_____

Major Defining Characteristics _____

_____

Minor Defining Characteristics _____

_____

NANDA _____

_____

Nursing Care Plan _____

_____

Nursing Diagnosis _____

_____

Nursing Process _____

_____

Objective Data _____

_____

Patient Goal _____

_____

Patient Outcome _____

_____

PES _____

_____

Planning _____

_____

Prioritize _____

_____

Qualifier _____

_____

Related Factors _____

_____

Risk Nursing Diagnosis _____

_____

Short-Term Outcome _____

_____

Subjective Data _____

_____

Taxonomy _____

_____

Wellness Nursing Diagnosis_____

_____

Laboratory Activities

1. Describe/define the *nursing process.*

   _____

   _____

   _____

   _____

   _____

2. What information is collected in the *assessment* phase of the nursing process?

   _____

   _____

   _____

   _____

   _____

3. Differentiate *subjective* and *objective* data.

   _____

   _____

   _____

   _____

   _____

4. Compare the approach of the *Body System Assessment* with the *Functional Health Patterns* assessment. Which approach is *cephalocaudal?*

   _____

   _____

   _____

   _____

   _____

5. Describe the three types of *nursing diagnoses* and give an example of each relating to the care of a patient with diabetes mellitus.

	Description	Example
Actual Nursing Diagnosis		
Risk Nursing Diagnosis		
Wellness Nursing Diagnosis		

6. What is the *PES* method for writing a nursing diagnosis?

_____

_____

_____

_____

_____

7. List five common errors in writing nursing diagnoses.
    (1) _____
    (2) _____
    (3) _____
    (4) _____
    (5) _____

8. What steps are involved in the *planning* phase of the nursing process? Why should the patient be involved in this phase?

_____

_____

_____

_____

9. What nursing actions are involved in the *implementation* phase of the nursing process?

_____

_____

_____

_____

10. How do *critical pathways* compare to the *nursing care plan*? Does *evaluation* differ in the two processes?

_____

_____

_____

_____

_____

Self-Assessment Quiz

1. What are the five phases of the nursing process?

    (1) _____

    (2) _____

    (3) _____

    (4) _____

    (5) _____

2. Match each of the following to the phase of the nursing process in which it occurs:

    _____ Patient's progress toward outcomes is determined

    _____ Time frame varies with each patient

    _____ Nursing database

    _____ Patient goals

    _____ Major and minor defining characteristics

    _____ Information based on *Functional Health Patterns*

    _____ Prioritization of nursing diagnoses

    _____ Helps patient meet predetermined outcomes

    _____ May review factors preventing goal achievement

    _____ Clinical judgment about patient responses to
    health problems

    A Assessment

    N Nursing Diagnosis

    P Planning

    I Implementation

    E Evaluation

3. **True or False?**

    ☐ **T** ☐ **F** *Maslow's Hierarchy of Needs* could be used to prioritize interventions.

    ☐ **T** ☐ **F** *Critical pathways* are based on the patient's *Diagnostic Related Grouping*.

    ☐ **T** ☐ **F** Short-term and long-term outcomes are included for every *patient outcome*.

    ☐ **T** ☐ **F** *Patient goals* should be well-defined with measurable outcomes.

    ☐ **T** ☐ **F** *Nursing diagnoses* are usually excluded from critical pathways.

    ☐ **T** ☐ **F** The third step of nursing diagnosis formulation is *clustering* of information.

    ☐ **T** ☐ **F** *Collaborative interventions* utilize resources from departments other than nursing.

4. Which of the following diagnoses are written incorrectly?

   A. Impaired adjustment related to necessity for major lifestyle change.
   B. Hyperemesis gravidarum related to abnormal fluid loss secondary to vomiting.
   C. Risk for injury related to altered clotting factors.
   D. Altered nutrition, more than body requirements, related to eating too much.

5. The _____ combines the elements of the nursing process to document the progress of patient care in a standardized fashion.

Lab Practice for The Patient Interview

Learning Objectives

1. Identify effective interviewing techniques.
2. Conduct a patient interview on your lab partner.
3. Describe characteristics of nontherapeutic and problematic interviewing techniques.
4. Identify interviewing techniques used with special populations.

Reading Assignment

Prior to beginning this lab assignment, please read Chapter 2, "The Patient Interview," in *Health Assessment & Physical Examination* by Mary Ellen Zator Estes, pages 17–38

Key Terms

Please define the following terms:

Action Response _____

_____

Active Listening _____

_____

Colloquialism _____

_____

Intermediary _____

_____

Joining Stage _____

_____

Listening Response _____

_____

Nonverbal Communication _____

_____

Termination Stage _____

_____

Working Stage _____

_____

Laboratory Activities

1. What types of information are collected during the patient interview?

   _____

   _____

   _____

   _____

   _____

2. How is the patient an active participant in the interview process?

   _____

   _____

   _____

   _____

   _____

3. Describe what occurs in each stage of the interview process:

   Stage I: *Joining* _____

   Stage II: *Working* _____

   Stage III: *Termination* _____

4. What role can family members or caregivers play during the interview process?

   _____

   _____

   _____

   _____

   _____

5. Give five examples of *nonverbal cues* that the nurse may observe.

   (1) _____

   (2) _____

   (3) _____

   (4) _____

   (5) _____

6. Contrast *listening responses* and *action responses* in the patient interview.

   _____

   _____

   _____

   _____

   _____

7. How much distance would each of the following represent in the United States?

*Personal distance*_____

Social distance _____

*Public distance*_____

Which is normally used for the patient interview?

_____

8. Give an example for each of these effective *questioning* and *listening response* techniques:

Open-ended question_____

Closed question _____

Making observations _____

Restating _____

Reflecting _____

Clarifying_____

Sequencing _____

Encouraging comparisons _____

Summarizing _____

How can silence be an effective tool?

_____

_____

_____

_____

_____

9. What *nontherapeutic* interviewing technique does each of the following statements represent?
Rewrite each for a more appropriate statement.

(1) "Why did you get pregnant again so soon?"

_____

_____

(2) "You don't want to take more pain medicine yet, do you?"

_____

_____

(3) "You won't have any trouble doing this dressing change at home."

_____

_____

(4) "If I were you, I'd definitely have that lump removed."

_____

_____

10. Contrast each of the following pairs of *effective vs. ineffective* techniques:

Exploring vs. probing_____

_____

Informing vs. advising _____

_____

Normalizing vs. false reassurance _____

_____

Limit setting vs. interrupting_____

_____

Presenting reality vs. defending _____

_____

11. What interviewing strategies may be helpful when confronted with a *hostile* patient?

_____

_____

_____

_____

_____

Signs of increasing tension in the patient may include:

_____

_____

_____

_____

_____

12. List three strategies to facilitate interviewing each of the following patients:

Hearing-impaired _____

_____

_____

Visually impaired _____

_____

_____

Aphasic _____

_____

_____

Non–English speaking _____

_____

_____

Low IQ_____

_____

_____

13. What special needs may the elderly patient have during the interview process?

_____

_____

_____

_____

_____

Self-Assessment Quiz

1. _____, or the act of perceiving what is said both verbally and nonverbally, is a critical factor in conducting a successful health assessment interview.

2. Identify five *problematic* questioning techniques.

    (1) _____

    (2) _____

    (3) _____

    (4) _____

    (5) _____

3. **True or False?**

    ☐ T ☐ F   Speaking more loudly and slowly to a patient who lip-reads is helpful.

    ☐ T ☐ F   *Social distance* allows for good eye contact.

    ☐ T ☐ F   Closed questions are best to use with the aphasic patient.

    ☐ T ☐ F   Ask permission before touching a visually impaired patient.

    ☐ T ☐ F   "Take a moment to get hold of yourself" allows an angry patient to refocus.

    ☐ T ☐ F   "You don't drink, do you?" is an example of *probing*.

4. What technique is used for each of the following statements?

    Reflecting   Collaborating

    Confronting   Informing

    Normalizing   Focusing

    Exploring   Encouraging comparisons

    _____ "Tell me more about the symptoms you experienced yesterday."

    _____ "You sound upset about that."

    _____ "You talked about your problems following the diet. Let's talk a little more about that."

    _____ "Have you had this type of headache before?"

    _____ "Many patients have the same concerns you do about this type of treatment."

5. Techniques to handle a *sexually aggressive* patient include:

_____

_____

_____

_____

_____

_____

Lab Practice for The Complete Health History

Chapter 3

Learning Objectives

1. Identify the components of a complete health history.
2. Complete a history of present illness (HPI) for a chief complaint.
3. Draw a genogram to illustrate a family health history.
4. Conduct a review of systems (ROS) on your lab partner.

Reading Assignment

Prior to beginning this lab assignment, please read Chapter 3, "The Complete Health History," in *Health Assessment & Physical Examination* by Mary Ellen Zator Estes, pages 39–67

Key Terms

Please define the following terms:

Aggravating Factors _____

_____

Alleviating Factors _____

_____

Associated Manifestations _____

_____

Cephalocaudal _____

_____

Characteristic Patterns of Daily Living _____

_____

Chief Complaint _____

_____

Complete Health History _____

_____

Distress _____

_____

Emergency Health History_____

_____

Episodic Health History _____

_____

Eustress _____

_____

Follow-Up Health History _____

_____

Genogram _____

_____

Health Maintenance Activities _____

_____

History of the Present Illness _____

_____

Interval (or Follow-Up) Health History _____

_____

Pack/Year History _____

_____

Past Health History _____

_____

Patient Profile _____

_____

Pertinent Negatives _____

_____

Reason for Seeking Health Care _____

_____

Review of Systems _____

_____

Sequelae _____

_____

Sign _____

_____

Social History _____

_____

Stress _____

_____

Symptom _____

_____

Visual Analog Scale _____

_____

Laboratory Activities

1. What are the purposes of a written health history? Why is the health history interview usually completed prior to the physical assessment?

    _____

    _____

    _____

    _____

    _____

    _____

2. In what situations might the source of the information be someone other than the patient?

    _____

    _____

    _____

    _____

    _____

3. What diseases would be noted in the *communicable disease* section?

    _____

    _____

    _____

    _____

    _____

    What diseases can be included in the *childhood illnesses* section?

    _____

    _____

    _____

    _____

    _____

4. What are the nine characteristics of a *chief complaint* that need to be included for a complete *history of present illness*?

    (1) _____

    (2) _____

    (3) _____

    (4) _____

    (5) _____

    (6) _____

    (7) _____

    (8) _____

    (9) _____

Suggest ways a patient could describe the severity of a symptom.

_____

_____

_____

_____

_____

5. List five questions that you might ask a patient for the *ROS* for each of the following:

Skin

(1) _____

(2) _____

(3) _____

(4) _____

(5) _____

Cardiovascular

(1) _____

(2) _____

(3) _____

(4) _____

(5) _____

Musculoskeletal

(1) _____

(2) _____

(3) _____

(4) _____

(5) _____

Female/Male Reproductive

(1) _____

(2) _____

(3) _____

(4) _____

(5) _____

6. Construct a genogram using information from your lab partner. Try to include the grandparents and any aunts and uncles.

7. You will now be conducting the first part of the health and physical assessment. Using your lab partner as a patient, conduct a complete health history for the following information:

Identifying Information

Today's Date _____

Biographical Data

Patient Name _____

Address _____

Phone Number _____

Date of Birth _____

Birthplace _____

Social Security Number _____

Occupation _____

Insurance _____

Usual Source of Health Care _____

Source of Referral _____

Emergency Contact _____

Complete Health History Assessment Tool

**Source and Reliability
of Information** _____

Patient Profile

Age _____

Sex _____

Race _____

Marital Status _____

**Reason for Seeking Health Care
or Chief Complaint** _____

**Present Health or
History of Present Illness**

Location _____

Radiation _____

Quality _____

Quantity _____

Associated Manifestations _____

Aggravating Factors _____

Alleviating Factors _____

Setting _____

Timing _____

Meaning and Impact _____

Past Health History

Medical History _____

_____

_____

Surgical History _____

_____

_____

Medications

   Prescription _____

_____

   Over-the-Counter _____

_____

   General Questions _____

Communicable Diseases _____

_____

Allergies _____

Injuries/Accidents _____

_____

Disabilities/Handicaps _____

Blood Transfusions _____

Childhood Illnesses _____

_____

Immunizations _____

_____

Family Health History _____

(Include a genogram.) _____

_____

Social History

Alcohol Use _____

Tobacco Use _____

Drug Use _____

Sexual Practice _____

Travel History _____

Work Environment _____

_____

Home Environment

   Physical Environment _____

_____

   Psychosocial Environment _____

Hobbies/Leisure Activities _____

_____

Stress _____

Education _____

Economic Status _____

Military Service _____

Religion _____

Ethnic Background _____

Roles/Relationships _____

Characteristic Patterns of

    Daily Living _____

_____

_____

_____

Health Maintenance Activities

Sleep _____

Diet _____

Exercise _____

Stress Management _____

Use of Safety Devices _____

_____

Health Check-ups

_____

_____

Review of Systems

General

_____

Neurological

_____

Psychological

_____

Skin

_____

Eyes

_____

Ears

_____

Nose and Sinuses

_____

Mouth

_____

Throat/Neck

_____

Respiratory

_____

Cardiovascular

_____

Breasts

_____

Gastrointestinal

_____

Urinary

_____

Musculoskeletal

_____

Female Reproductive

_____

Male Reproductive

_____

Nutrition

_____

Endocrine

_____

Lymph Nodes

_____

_____

Hematological

_____

_____

8. How can you deal with sensitive topics such as alcohol use, drug use, or sexual practices during the health history?

_____

_____

_____

_____

_____

Self-Assessment Quiz

1. What are the four types of health history?
   (1) _____
   (2) _____
   (3) _____
   (4) _____

2. In which section of the health history would each of these items be noted?

   _____ Denies hx of hepatitis, AIDS

   _____ Works long hours at stressful job

   _____ College graduate

   _____ Denies change in moles

   _____ Husband is emergency contact

   _____ Asian

   _____ Felt "well" until two days ago

   _____ Sibling died in skiing accident

   _____ "I have an itchy rash on my legs."

   _____ Drinks beer to relax

   _____ Blood type "O Negative"

   A. Biographical Data

   B. Patient Profile

   C. Chief Complaint

   D. History of Present Illness

   E. Past Health History

   F. Family Health History

   G. Social History

   H. Health Maintenance Activities

   I. Review of Systems

3. True or False?

   ☐ **T** ☐ **F** Terms such as "burning," "stabbing," and "aching" describe the *quantity* of pain.

   ☐ **T** ☐ **F** A *sign* is an objective finding; a *symptom* is a subjective finding.

   ☐ **T** ☐ **F** Information on the *setting* for a CC can include the patient's mental state.

   ☐ **T** ☐ **F** Exposure to communicable diseases is usually limited to the last ten years.

   ☐ **T** ☐ **F** A well-drawn genogram eliminates the need for a list of familial diseases.

   ☐ **T** ☐ **F** The ROS usually follows a cephalocaudal approach.

   ☐ **T** ☐ **F** Questions about sexual practice should be omitted on the patient's first visit.

4. "What's missing from this picture?" Read this HPI in the patient's own words, and decide which of the nine characteristics of a chief complaint are missing.

CC: *"I have a swollen ankle."*

HPI: *"About three weeks ago, I hurt the inside of my left ankle on the edge of a desk and it's been swollen and sore off and on since then. It gets a little achy if I try to walk too far at one time, or if I try to jog on it, so I've given that up for now. I tried some of that sports tape wrapped around it, and that helped, but I'm just getting tired of having it like this. You know, I'd like to go jogging again before the weather gets too cold."*

The missing characteristics are: _____

_____

5. Draw a *genogram* using the following information. (Add any abbreviations used in the genogram to the legend.)

Patient is female, married, 21 years old, and has mild asthma.

Her husband is 23 and alive and well.

They have a 2-year-old son who is a little obnoxious, but alive and well.

Her parents are both 49 years old, divorced. Her father has hypertension and her mother has migraine headaches.

She has two brothers, a 26-year-old who is alive and well and one who died in a motor vehicle accident at the age of 19.

Her maternal grandparents include her 75-year-old grandmother, with congestive heart failure, and her grandfather, who died at the age of 68 of a myocardial infarction.

There is no information on her paternal grandparents or any aunts or uncles.

LEGEND

◯ Living female

☐ Living male

● or ⊗ Deceased female

■ or ◻ Deceased male

⟋ Points to patient

◯◯ Female twins

☐☐ Male twins

—‖— or ----- Divorced

A&W = Alive & well

CA = Cancer

HTN = Hypertension

Lab Practice for Developmental Assessment

Chapter 4

Learning Objectives

1. Compare growth and developmental theories.
2. Describe developmental assessment tools.
3. Identify the current stage of development for your lab partner.
4. Conduct developmental assessments on patients of different ages.

Reading Assignment

Prior to beginning this lab assignment, please read Chapter 4, "Developmental Assessment," in *Health Assessment & Physical Examination* by Mary Ellen Zator Estes, pages 71–99.

Key Terms

Please define the following terms:

Ages and Stages Developmental Theory _____

_____

Castration Anxiety _____

_____

Conservation _____

_____

Development _____

_____

Developmental Stage _____

_____

Developmental Task _____

_____

Ego _____

_____

Egocentrism _____

_____

Electra Complex _____

_____

Growth _____

_____

Id _____

_____

Life Event/Transitional Developmental Theory _____

_____

Life Review _____

_____

Object Permanence _____

_____

Oedipus Complex_____

_____

Penis Envy _____

_____

Reversibility _____

_____

Superego _____

_____

Laboratory Activities

1. Differentiate *growth* from *development*.

_____

_____

_____

_____

_____

2. Compare the *ages and stages* theory of development to the *life events/transitional* theory.

_____

_____

_____

_____

_____

Name four theorists who have generated *ages and stages* development theories.

(1) _____

(2) _____

(3) _____

(4) _____

3. What are *cognitive life skills* in Piaget's theory of cognitive development?

_____

_____

_____

_____

_____

List the four stages of Piaget's theory of development and the major tasks of each.

Developmental Stage	Major Tasks

4. Differentiate the concepts of the *id*, the *ego*, and the *superego* according to Freud.

_____

_____

_____

_____

_____

5. Identify the age and major conflicts for each of Freud's *psychosexual stages* of development.

Stage	Age Range	Major Conflicts
Oral		
Anal		
Phallic		
Latency		
Genital		

6. What are the eight stages in Erikson's theory of personality development?

(1) _____

(2) _____

(3) _____

(4) _____

(5) _____

(6) _____

(7) _____

(8) _____

How do individuals progress from one stage to the next?

_____

_____

_____

_____

_____

What stage do you feel correlates with your lab partner, and why?

_____

_____

_____

_____

_____

_____

7. What are the three levels of Kohlberg's *theory of moral development*?

(1) _____

(2) _____

(3) _____

8. Compare the following theorists' views of the stages of development for an individual at ages 5, 15, and 25:

	Age 5	Age 15	Age 25
Freud			
Piaget			
Erikson			
Kohlberg			

9. Describe the purpose of each of the following developmental assessment tools:

Tool	Purpose
Brazelton Neonatal Behavioral Assessment Scale	
Denver II	
Early Language Milestones Scale	
Modified Erikson Psychosocial Stage Inventory	
Life Experiences Survey	
Stress Audit	
Functional Activities Questionnaire	
Minimum Data Set for Nursing Facility Resident Assessment and Care Screening	
Folstein Mini-Mental State Examination	
Beck Depression Inventory	

Which tools can be self-administered or used by a caregiver?

_____

_____

_____

_____

_____

10. Which of the developmental assessment tools (refer to pp. 90–94 in your text) would help determine the developmental level of a preschooler?

_____

_____

_____

_____

_____

11. What information can be obtained from the *Recent Life Changes Questionnaire?*

_____

_____

_____

_____

_____

Conduct the *Recent Life Changes Questionnaire* on yourself and your lab partner (refer to pp. 94–97 in your text).

What are your total life stress scores?

_____

_____

_____

_____

What conclusions might you draw from your results?

_____

_____

_____

_____

Self-Assessment Quiz

1. The most frequently used theory of personality development is _____.

2. In which development stage would these life events most likely occur?

_____ Getting married

_____ Beginning menopause

_____ Developing a conscience

_____ Developing a basic sense of trust

_____ Beginning self-care (feeding, dressing)

_____ Adopting moral standards for behavior

_____ Adjusting to rapid physical and sexual changes

3. **True or False?**

   ☐ **T** ☐ **F**   Ages 55 to 70 are considered *middle adulthood*.

   ☐ **T** ☐ **F**   The *Minimum Data Set* (MDS) is required by law for nursing home residents.

   ☐ **T** ☐ **F**   *Egocentrism* is a characterization of Piaget's sensorimotor stage.

   ☐ **T** ☐ **F**   The *Denver II* is the most widely used developmental screening tool.

   ☐ **T** ☐ **F**   Moral development (Kohlberg) parallels cognitive behavior development.

   ☐ **T** ☐ **F**   Chronic diseases are often first diagnosed in *early middle adulthood*.

4. **Match the following terms and descriptions.**

   _____ Profiles personal-social, fine motor-adaptive, language, and gross motor skills

   _____ Predicts susceptibility to stress-related illness

   _____ Identifies children with attention deficit disorders

   _____ Assesses level of independence in performing ADLs

   _____ Most widely used test of cognitive function in the elderly

   _____ Tests comprehensibility, manageability, and meaningfulness

   A. Folstein MMSE

   B. Sense of Coherence Scale

   C. Functional Activities Questionnaire

   D. Denver II

   E. ACTeRS Scale

   F. Recent Life Changes Questionnaire

5. A _____ allows the elderly to evaluate their experiences, relationships, successes, and failures from the perspective of age.

Lab Practice for Cultural Assessment

Learning Objectives

1. Compare characteristics of various cultures.
2. Identify components of a cultural assessment.
3. Conduct a comprehensive cultural assessment on your lab partner or patient.
4. Identify cultural influences on health values and behaviors.

Reading Assignment

Prior to beginning this lab assignment, please read Chapter 5, "Cultural Assessment," in *Health Assessment & Physical Examination* by Mary Ellen Zator Estes, pages 101–127.

Key Terms

Please define the following terms:

Acculturation _____

_____

Bilingualism_____

_____

Cross-Cultural Nursing Care _____

_____

Cultural Beliefs _____

_____

Cultural Diversity _____

_____

Cultural Identity _____

_____

Cultural Norms _____

_____

Cultural Relativism _____

_____

Cultural Rituals _____

_____

Cultural Values _____

_____

Culturally Competent Nursing Care _____

_____

Culture_____

_____

Culture Shock _____

_____

Custom _____

_____

Ecogram_____

_____

Enculturation _____

_____

Ethnic Group _____

_____

Ethnic Identity _____

_____

Ethnocentrism _____

_____

Folk Illness _____

_____

Folk Practitioner _____

_____

Minority Group Members _____

_____

Multicultural Identity _____

_____

Multiculturalism _____

_____

Naturalistic Illness _____

_____

Personalistic Illness _____

_____

Race _____

_____

Scientific Illness _____

_____

Subculture_____

_____

Value Orientation _____

_____

Laboratory Activities

1. Describe *culturally competent* nursing care.

   _____

   _____

   _____

   _____

   _____

2. Contrast *racial* and *ethnic* groups.

   _____

   _____

   _____

   _____

   _____

   What are the five ethnic groups usually recognized in the United States?

   (1) _____

   (2) _____

   (3) _____

   (4) _____

   (5) _____

3. Why is it appropriate to determine an individual's place of birth as well as his self-identified ethnic group?

   _____

   _____

   _____

   _____

   _____

4. Identify your own *primary culture* and the *subcultures* of which you are a member.

   _____

   _____

   _____

   _____

   Does your lab partner identify with a different primary culture and subcultures?

   _____

   _____

   _____

   _____

5. How does your lab partner view each of the following *values*?

<u>   **Value Orientation and Beliefs**   </u>

Time: What is the time orientation
of human beings?

_____

Human Nature: What is the basic
nature of human beings?

_____

Activity: What is the primary purpose
of life?

_____

Relational: What is the purpose of human
relations?

_____

People to Nature: What is the relationship
of human beings to nature?

_____

How do your own value orientation and beliefs differ from those of your lab partner?

_____

_____

_____

_____

_____

6. Differentiate *customs* and *cultural rituals*.

_____

_____

_____

_____

_____

7. Compare the following characteristics of *family* and *kinship patterns*:

Characteristics	Cultural Groups
Linear	
Collateral	
Individualistic	

8. What is the importance of self-care practices and home remedies to a patient?

9. Using your lab partner as a patient, follow the *Culturally Competent Assessment Guide* questionnaire (beginning on p. 123 in your text) to summarize the following information:

Ethnic Group/Racial Background
How long have you lived here?
Primary ethnic group?
How closely do you identify with
this group?
Exposure to health problems?

Major Beliefs and Values
What traditions and beliefs are related
to your health practices?

Health Beliefs and Practices
What does it mean to be healthy or
sick?
What do you do when you are sick?
Whom do you prefer to provide
health care?

Language Barriers and Communication Styles
What language do you prefer?
Need an interpreter for health care?
Cultural preferences for social contact?

Role of Family, Spousal Relationship, Parenting Styles

Ethnic background of your family? _____

Who are members of your family? _____

How can health care workers help you
achieve health and well-being? _____

10. Contrast *naturalistic* illnesses and *personalistic* illnesses.

_____

_____

_____

Which cultures share the *evil eye* belief?

_____

_____

_____

11. According to Korbin, a child-rearing practice of a particular culture would not be perceived as
harmful under the following five conditions:

(1) _____

(2) _____

(3) _____

(4) _____

(5) _____

12. List one health value or custom that might have a *positive* influence and one that might have a
negative influence on medical treatment for each of the following cultural groups:

Cultural Group	Possible Positive Influence	Possible Negative Influence
Asian-American		
African-American		
Hispanic American		
American Indian		
Middle Eastern		
White American		

Self-Assessment Quiz

1. _____ is a learned and socially transmitted orientation and way of life of a group of people.

2. True or False?

   ☐ T ☐ F   The fastest-growing minority in the United States is Hispanic.

   ☐ T ☐ F   A diagram of an individual's relationships to family, friends, peers, and neighbors is called a sociogram.

   ☐ T ☐ F   Communication variables include eye contact, topic taboos, and who makes health care decisions in the family.

   ☐ T ☐ F   Asian, Middle Eastern, and Hispanic families are typically patriarchal.

   ☐ T ☐ F   Behaviors associated with healing, marriage, and worship are examples of values.

   ☐ T ☐ F   Cultural relativism is a belief that no culture is superior to another.

   ☐ T ☐ F   All cultural groups use self-care practices.

3. In 1990, the population of the United States was:

   _____ % Euro-American

   _____ % African-American

   _____ % Hispanic

   _____ % Asian

   _____ % American Indian

4. An informal process of adaptation to a dominant culture by new members from another culture is called _____.

   Disorientation, uncertainty, and alienation that can occur during the process of adjusting is called _____.

5. Match the following cultural groups and characteristics.

_____ Folk care practices include *cao gio* (rubbing skin with coin) and *bat gil* (skin pinching)	A. Haitian
_____ Health results from a balance between energy forces *yin* (cold) and *yang* (hot)	B. American Indian
_____ Use folk practices "first and last"	C. Middle Eastern
_____ May use herbalists, midwives, or voodoo priests	D. African-American
_____ Prevent and treat illness with "hot" and "cold" food prescriptions and prohibitions	E. Mexican
_____ Prayer a common means for prevention and treatment of illness	F. Chinese
_____ May use a medicine man, diviner-diagnostician, and singers to help with illness	G. Appalachian
_____ Emotional distress may be expressed as "heart disease"	H. Vietnamese

Lab Practice for Spiritual Assessment

Learning Objectives

1. Identify and compare characteristics of religious beliefs.
2. Conduct a spiritual assessment on your lab partner.
3. Identify signs that indicate a patient is experiencing spiritual distress.
4. Determine appropriate interactions with patients in spiritual distress.

Reading Assignment

Prior to beginning this lab assignment, please read Chapter 6, "Spiritual Assessment," in *Health Assessment & Physical Examination* by Mary Ellen Zator Estes, pages 129–152.

Key Terms

Please define the following terms:

Advance Directive _____

_____

Agnostic_____

_____

Animism _____

_____

Atheist _____

_____

Code of Ethics_____

_____

Cult _____

_____

Dogma _____

_____

Faith_____

_____

God _____

_____

Heaven_____

_____

Heretic _____

Holistic Nursing _____

Monotheism _____

Nirvana _____

Pagan _____

Pastoral Care _____

Polytheism _____

Prayer _____

Reincarnation _____

Religion _____

Ritual _____

Schismatic _____

Sin _____

Soul _____

Spirit _____

Spiritual Distress _____

Spiritual Well-Being _____

Spirituality _____

Laboratory Activities

1. Spiritual support may be helpful during times of change or crisis, such as:

   _____

   _____

   _____

   _____

   _____

2. Contrast *spirituality* and *religion*.

   _____

   _____

   _____

   _____

   _____

3. What information is included in the *spiritual assessment*?

   _____

   _____

   _____

   _____

   _____

4. What are signs that a patient may be experiencing *spiritual distress*?

   _____

   _____

   _____

   _____

   _____

5. Using your lab partner as a patient, conduct a spiritual assessment, beginning with the following questions:

   (1) Do you have an advance directive (Living Will or Durable Medical Power of Attorney)?_____

   _____

   (2) Have you signed an organ donor card or thought about donating any organs or tissue after death?_____

   _____

   (3) Do you hold any spiritual or religious beliefs that will affect your health care? _____

   _____

   (4) (Have you noted any outward signs such as religious clothing or jewelry that may relate to the spiritual beliefs of the patient?) _____

   _____

(5) Who should be notified if there is a change in your condition? _____

_____

(6) Do you want me to notify a place of worship or a specific religious leader? _____

_____

(7) Additional information or observations: _____

_____

6. What nursing interventions are appropriate for the patient in spiritual distress?

_____

_____

_____

_____

_____

7. What type of support can a hospital chaplain provide for the patient?

_____

_____

_____

_____

_____

8. Actions or statements you should *avoid* when intervening in the patient's spiritual condition include:

_____

_____

_____

_____

_____

Why are clichés inappropriate?

_____

_____

_____

_____

_____

9. What are signs that a patient may exhibit when spiritual distress has *decreased*?

_____

_____

_____

_____

_____

Self-Assessment Quiz

1. What are two NANDA nursing diagnoses that address the spiritual care of the patient?

   (1) _____

   (2) _____

2. **True or False?**

   □ **T** □ **F** The spiritual assessment is better if conducted as a stand-alone interview.

   □ **T** □ **F** Spiritual beliefs help the patient define her ultimate purpose in life.

   □ **T** □ **F** Choosing a quiet, private room with dim lighting will help the assessment.

   □ **T** □ **F** Hinduism is an example of a monotheistic religion.

   □ **T** □ **F** Nursing interventions attempt to resolve spiritual distress.

   □ **T** □ **F** Hospitals are required to conduct a spiritual history on all inpatients.

   □ **T** □ **F** The question "What is your religion?" may be inappropriate.

3. Fill in the blanks:

   A. For some patients, _____ is an essential ingredient in health care.

   B. _____ is the belief that after death, the person lives another life on earth in another body.

   C. _____ refers to the essential beliefs at the core of a religion.

   D. _____ is the belief that all things in nature have a soul.

   E. Birth, accidents, illness, and dying all can provoke _____ in a patient.

4. The statement "It'll all look better tomorrow" is an example of a _____.

   The statement "It was God's will" is an example of a _____.

5. In which religion are these found? (Some may have more than one answer.)

_____ Generally against donating or receiving organs	**A** American Indian
_____ Illness may be related to sin, an unhappy spirit, or god	**B** Buddhism
_____ Life support seen as unnatural and unnecessary	**H** Hinduism
_____ Organ donation permitted	**I** Islam
_____ Holy water poured into the mouth of a dying person	**J** Judaism
_____ Birth control and infertility treatment permitted	**P** Protestant
_____ Complex dietary rules not observed by all members	**R** Roman Catholic/ Orthodox
_____ Good karma results from saving, prolonging, or improving life	
_____ Pork and pork products, alcohol and street drugs are forbidden	
_____ Anointing of the sick with oil and prayers may be done often during an illness	

_____ Privacy should be maintained for females during hospitalization, with long-sleeved gowns if possible

_____ After death, the body should not be disturbed with movement, talking, or crying

_____ Healing the sick considered the highest service to God, after religious requirements

_____ Many prefer to die as close to mother earth as possible, even on the floor or ground

Lab Practice for Nutritional Assessment

Chapter 7

Learning Objectives

1. Describe dietary guidelines from the Food Guide Pyramid.
2. Conduct a nutritional screening on your lab partner.
3. Complete a comprehensive nutritional assessment on your lab partner.
4. Evaluate subjective and objective data to determine nutritional status.
5. Identify abnormal patterns of nutrition and diseases.

Reading Assignment

Prior to beginning this lab assignment, please read Chapter 7, "Nutritional Assessment," in *Health Assessment & Physical Examination* by Mary Ellen Zator Estes, pages 153–184.

Key Terms

Please define the following terms:

Albumin _____

_____

Anergy _____

_____

Anthropometric Measurements _____

_____

Anticipatory Guidance _____

_____

Antigen Skin Testing _____

_____

Atherosclerosis _____

_____

Cachexia _____

_____

Carbohydrate _____

_____

Cholesterol _____

_____

Creatinine _____
_____

Fats_____
_____

Fat-Soluble Vitamins _____
_____

Food Guide Pyramid_____
_____

Hematocrit _____
_____

Hemoglobin _____
_____

High-Density Lipoprotein _____
_____

Hyperglycemia _____
_____

Hypoglycemia _____
_____

Kilocalorie_____
_____

Kwashiorkor _____
_____

Low-Density Lipoprotein _____
_____

Macromineral _____
_____

Marasmus_____
_____

Micromineral_____
_____

Mid-Arm Circumference_____
_____

Mid-Arm Muscle Circumference _____
_____

Mineral_____
_____

Monosaturated Fats _____
_____

Nitrogen _____
_____

Nutrient _____

_____

Nutrition _____

_____

Obesity _____

_____

Osteoporosis _____

_____

Pica _____

_____

Proteins _____

_____

Recommended Dietary Allowance _____

_____

Saturated Fats _____

_____

Serum Iron _____

_____

Skinfold Thickness _____

_____

Total Iron-Binding Capacity _____

_____

Transferrin _____

_____

Triceps Skinfold _____

_____

Triglyceride _____

_____

Vitamin _____

_____

Water-Soluble Vitamin _____

_____

Laboratory Activities

1. List the food groups and recommended number of servings for adults from the *Food Guide Pyramid.*

Food Group	Number of Servings

2. In what ways have the dietary guidelines (the Food Guide Pyramid) changed from the *Basic Four* food guidelines issued in 1956?

_____

_____

_____

_____

3. Each age group has special physical and psychological characteristics that can affect its nutritional status. What are some of these characteristics, and what suggestions could you offer patients to maintain a healthy nutritional status?

Age Group	Characteristics	Suggestions
Infants		
Toddlers		
Preschoolers		

Age Group	Characteristics	Suggestions
School-age children		
Adolescents		
Young and middle-aged adults		
Pregnant/lactating women		

4. What are the signs and symptoms of *dehydration*?

_____

_____

_____

_____

_____

5. **ROS (Review of Systems).** Ask your lab partner the following questions:

_____

Do you have any concerns about your diet or eating?

_____

Any change in weight?

_____

Any change in appetite or dietary habits?

_____

Any difficulty with feeding yourself, eating, chewing or swallowing?

_____

Any nausea, vomiting, diarrhea, or constipation?

_____

What are your food likes and dislikes? Any cravings?

_____

How do you prepare and store food?

_____

Eat alone or with others?

_____

Take vitamins, supplements, or liquid diets?

_____

Follow a particular diet?

_____

Family hx of obesity, high cholesterol, diabetes, CAD, HTN, CA, or CVA?

_____

Any fatigue, weakness, or frequent infections?

_____

Change in skin, nails, or hair?

_____

Any mouth sores?

_____

Any vision changes or eye discharge?

_____

Any headaches, irritability, or numbness?

_____

Pain, cramping, or frequent fractures?

_____

Any change in menstrual pattern?

_____

6. **Physical Exam.** (*Equipment: Scale with right-angle headboard, tape measure, skinfold calipers.*) Using your lab partner as a patient, follow the physical assessment guidelines (beginning on p. 173 of your text) to complete the following information:

Physical Assessment
(Refer to Table 7-8 in your text.)

General Appearance	_____
Skin, Hair, Nails	_____
Eyes	_____
Mouth	_____
Head and Neck	_____
Heart and Peripheral Vasculature	_____
Abdomen	_____
Musculoskeletal System	_____

Neurological System   _____

Female Genitalia   _____

Anthropometric Measurements

Height   _____

Weight   _____

Skinfold Thickness   _____

Mid-Arm Circumference   _____

Mid-Arm Muscle Circumference   _____

Laboratory Data (optional)

Hematocrit/Hemoglobin   _____

Cholesterol and Triglycerides   _____

Transferrin, Total Iron-Binding
   Capacity, and Iron   _____

Total Lymphocyte Count   _____

Antigen Skin Testing   _____

Albumin   _____

Glucose   _____

Creatinine Height Index   _____

Nitrogen Balance   _____

Diagnostic Data   _____

_____

7. Determine the *anthropometric measurements* for your lab partner. (Refer to Table 7-7 in your text.)

Height: _____

Weight: _____

$$\text{\% Ideal Body Weight} = \frac{\text{Current Weight}}{\text{IBW}} \times 100 = \underline{\hspace{2cm}}$$

$$\text{\% Usual Body Weight} = \frac{\text{Current Weight}}{\text{Usual Body Weight}} \times 100 = \underline{\hspace{2cm}}$$

$$\text{\% Weight Change} = \frac{\text{Usual Weight} - \text{Current Weight}}{\text{Usual Weight}} \times 100 = \underline{\hspace{2cm}}$$

Triceps Skinfold (TSF) _____ mm

Mid-Arm Circumference (MAC) _____ cm

Mid-Arm Muscle Circumference (MAMC)

     MAMC (cm) = MAC (cm) − [3.14 × TSF (cm)] = _____

What percentile is your lab partner's TSF, MAC, and MAMC?

_____

_____

_____

_____

_____

What do your findings indicate for your lab partner?

_____

_____

_____

_____

_____

8. An 18-year-old female's TSF is 8 mm. Her MAC is 230 mm. Calculate her MAMC.

_____

_____

_____

_____

_____

What nutritional recommendations could you offer?

_____

_____

_____

_____

_____

9. List five signs and symptoms of poor nutritional status in both the skin and the mouth.
   (1) _____
   (2) _____
   (3) _____
   (4) _____
   (5) _____

10. List the risk factors for osteoporosis.

_____

_____

_____

_____

_____

11. What differences would you note in laboratory data for *marasmus* and *kwashiorkor*?

	Marasmus	**Kwashiorkor**
TSF, MAC		
Weight		
Albumin		
Immune function		

12. What nutritional difficulties often arise in the aging population?

13. How can you individualize the recommendations from the Food Guide Pyramid to meet the special needs of the aging population?

Self-Assessment Quiz

1. As part of a complete nutritional assessment, *anticipatory guidance* includes:

2. Match these diseases with their findings:

_____ Deficiency of vitamin C

_____ Reduced bone mass

_____ Softening and deformities of the bones

_____ Affects primarily infants

_____ Occurs most often in children ages one to four

_____ Shows compensatory behavior to avoid weight gain

_____ Involves non-food cravings

_____ Includes amenorrhea

_____ Body weight less than 85% of expected weight

_____ Deficiency of vitamin D

_____ Risk factors include family hx and estrogen deficiency

A. Kwashiorkor

B. Marasmus

C. Anorexia nervosa

D. Bulimia nervosa

E. Osteoporosis

F. Pica

G. Scurvy

H. Rickets

3. Label the food groups in this diagram of the Food Guide Pyramid.

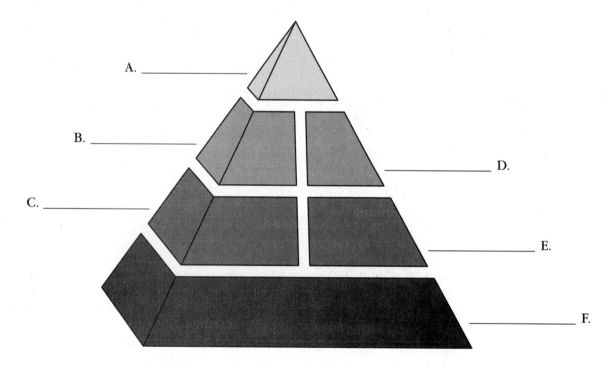

4. Which of the following patients would cause you the most concern?

Patient A: A 3-year-old seems to be eating less than his younger brother. He enjoys fruit juices and milk, but has shown a decline in his previously rapid growth rate. He often refuses to eat more than just one food at a meal.

Patient B: A 17-year-old female spends much of her time looking in the mirror and feels she probably doesn't look as good as her classmates. She has become more physically active and occasionally skips meals.

Patient C: A new mother who is breastfeeding her baby happily reports her loss of several pounds of "baby fat" since the birth one month ago. She reports eating a "good diet," with 8 ounces of juice or water four times a day.

Patient D: A 75-year-old patient who lives alone, but has family nearby, has been eating a little less and feels constipated at times. Her dentures don't fit as well any more. She tells her family she doesn't eat as much because "I can't taste it, anyway."

_____

_____

_____

_____

_____

5. Fill in the blanks:

   A. Water is essential to life and accounts for _____% of the body's weight.

   B. *Obesity* is defined as a weight greater than _____% of the ideal body weight.

   C. Protein should account for _____% of the diet for an adult.

   D. Over _____% of patients with *anorexia nervosa* are female.

6. **Bonus Question!** The first question to your patient regarding nutrition should *always* be:

   _____

   (*Hint:* It's not "What's for dessert?")

Lab Practice for Physical Assessment Techniques

Learning Objectives

1. Practice physical assessment techniques.
2. Identify and describe characteristics of percussion sounds.
3. Establish a systematic order for assessment procedures.
4. Demonstrate patient positioning and draping techniques.

Reading Assignment

Prior to beginning this lab assignment, please read Chapter 8, "Physical Assessment Techniques," in *Health Assessment & Physical Examination* by Mary Ellen Zator Estes, pages 189–202.

Key Terms

Please define the following terms:

Auscultation _____

_____

Deep Palpation _____

_____

Direct (or Immediate) Auscultation _____

_____

Direct Fist Percussion_____

_____

Direct (or Immediate) Percussion_____

_____

Dullness_____

_____

Duration (of Percussion) _____

_____

Flatness _____

_____

Hyperresonance _____

_____

Immediate Auscultation _____

_____

Immediate Percussion _____

_____

Indirect (or Mediate) Auscultation _____

_____

Indirect Fist Percussion _____

_____

Indirect (or Mediate) Percussion_____

_____

Inspection _____

_____

Intensity (of Percussion) _____

_____

Light Palpation _____

_____

Mediate Auscultation _____

_____

Mediate Percussion_____

_____

Palpation _____

_____

Percussion_____

_____

Pitch (of Percussion) _____

_____

Pleximeter_____

_____

Plexor _____

_____

Quality (of Percussion) _____

_____

Resonance_____

_____

Standard Precautions _____

_____

Tangential Lighting_____

_____

Tympany _____

_____

Laboratory Activities

1. Which part of your hand is most useful in assessing each of the following:

   Temperature _____

   Vibration _____

   Masses _____

   Edema _____

   Pulsations _____

   Fine tactile discrimination _____

2. Assist your lab partner into each of the following positions for patient examination (refer to p. 201 in your text). Use a drape as appropriate.

Semi-Fowler's	Side lying
High Fowler's	Lithotomy
Horizontal recumbent	Knee-chest
Dorsal recumbent	Sims'

3. What is the difference between *light* and *deep palpation*?

   _____

   _____

   _____

   _____

   _____

4. Practice the technique of *indirect percussion* on your lab partner to elicit different sounds (refer to p. 196 in your text). What sounds are produced over each of the following?

   Gastric bubble_____

   Lungs _____

   Muscle/bones _____

   Liver (organs) _____

5. Complete the following chart on the characteristics of percussion sounds:

	Location	Intensity	Duration	Pitch	Quality
Tympany					
Hyperresonance					
Resonance					
Dullness					
Flatness					

6. Percuss the frontal and maxillary sinuses with *immediate/direct percussion* and the kidneys with *mediate/indirect fist percussion*. Do you note any tenderness?

_____

_____

_____

_____

_____

7. In what order do you usually perform these physical assessment techniques?

_____ Palpation

_____ Auscultation

_____ Inspection

_____ Percussion

How does this pattern change for assessing the abdomen?

_____

_____

_____

_____

_____

8. Which *standard precautions* would you apply while assessing each of these patients?

A patient with *tuberculosis*: _____

_____

A patient with a wound infected with *Pseudomonas*:_____

_____

A patient with *Hepatitis A*: _____

_____

Self-Assessment Quiz

1. Name the four different types of percussion.

   (1) _____

   (2) _____

   (3) _____

   (4) _____

   Which is the preferred method for kidney assessment?

   _____

   _____

   _____

   _____

   _____

   _____

2. **True or False?**

   ☐ **T** ☐ **F**   Use the diaphragm of the stethoscope to listen for bruits and murmurs.

   ☐ **T** ☐ **F**   Hold the bell firmly on the skin surface to be auscultated.

   ☐ **T** ☐ **F**   Always conduct an assessment in a systematic fashion.

   ☐ **T** ☐ **F**   Frequency (or *pitch*) is caused by a sound's vibrations.

   ☐ **T** ☐ **F**   Earpieces on the stethoscope should point slightly away from the nose.

   ☐ **T** ☐ **F**   The bell transmits low-pitched sounds.

   ☐ **T** ☐ **F**   The most important aspect of infection control is the consistent and proper use of gloves.

3. Name each of the following positions:

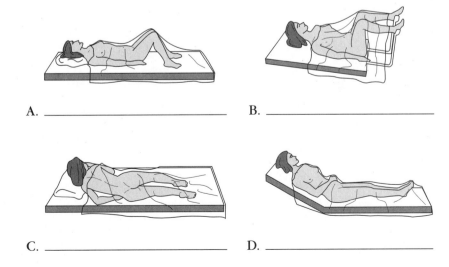

   A. _____   B. _____

   C. _____   D. _____

4. Match the following sounds:

_____ Predominant sound over the abdomen   A. Flat

_____ May indicate emphysema   B. Dull

_____ Heard over bone or muscle
                                                     C. Resonant
_____ Has a "hollow" quality

_____ Noted over the liver   D. Hyperresonant

_____ The sound with the shortest duration   E. Tympany

_____ The predominant sound over the lungs

5. What are the four main purposes of a physical assessment?

(1) _____

(2) _____

(3) _____

(4) _____

Lab Practice for General Assessment and Vital Signs

Chapter 9

Learning Objectives

1. Demonstrate a general assessment, including physical and psychological presence and any distress.
2. Assess vital signs using proper equipment and techniques.
3. Locate anatomical sites for pulse assessment.
4. Describe factors affecting vital sign measurement.
5. Identify normal and abnormal findings in general assessment and vital signs.

Reading Assignment

Prior to beginning this lab assignment, please read Chapter 9, "General Assessment and Vital Signs," in *Health Assessment & Physical Examination* by Mary Ellen Zator Estes, page 203–220.

Key Terms

Please define the following terms:

Aneroid Manometer _____

_____

Apnea _____

_____

Arrhythmia _____

_____

Asystole _____

_____

Baroreceptors _____

_____

Blood Pressure _____

_____

Bradycardia _____

_____

Bradypnea _____

_____

Circadian Rhythm _____

_____

Diastole _____

_____

Dysrhythmia _____

_____

Hypertension _____

_____

Hyperthermia _____

_____

Hypotension _____

_____

Hypothermia_____

_____

Korotkoff Sounds _____

_____

Mercury Manometer_____

_____

Peripheral Vascular Resistance _____

_____

Pulse _____

_____

Pulse Deficit _____

_____

Pulse Pressure_____

_____

Respiration _____

_____

Sphygmomanometer _____

_____

Systemic Vascular Resistance_____

_____

Systole _____

_____

Tachycardia _____

_____

Tachypnea _____

_____

Temperature _____

_____

Vital Signs _____

_____

Laboratory Activities

1. Blood pressure cuffs come in several sizes. How do you determine the correct size for your patient?

    _____

    _____

    _____

    _____

    _____

2. Try to locate all pulses on your lab partner (see p. 209 of your text).

Temporal	Brachial	Popliteal
Carotid	Radial	Posterior tibial
Apical	Femoral	Dorsalis pedis

3. How do you convert degrees of temperature:

    From Celsius to Fahrenheit? _____

    From Fahrenheit to Celsius? _____

4. Name one advantage and one disadvantage for each of these four basic routes for measuring body temperature:

	Advantage	Disadvantage
Oral		
Rectal		
Axillary		
Tympanic		

5. Complete this 4-point scale for measuring *pulse volume*:

_____

+0

_____

+1

_____

+2

_____

+3

_____

+4

_____

How does this 4-point scale compare with the 3-point scale?

_____
_____
_____
_____
_____

6. **Physical Exam.** *(Equipment: Stethoscope, watch with a second hand, thermometer, sphygmo-manometer.)* Using your lab partner as a patient, follow the physical assessment guidelines (beginning on p. 204 in your text) to complete the following information:

General Assessment

Physical presence

   Stated age versus apparent age   _____

   Body fat   _____

   Stature   _____

   Motor activity   _____

   Body and breath odors   _____

Psychological presence

   Dress, grooming, and personal

     hygiene   _____

   Mood and manner   _____

   Speech   _____

   Facial expression   _____

Distress   _____

Vital Signs

Respiration _____

Pulse _____

Temperature _____

Blood pressure _____

7. What can cause each of the following errors in blood pressure measurement?

   Inaccurately high BP _____

   High diastolic BP_____

   Inaccurately low BP _____

   Low systolic BP_____ .

8. Name three conditions that can cause a patient to have severe body or breath odors.

   (1) _____

   (2) _____

   (3) _____

9. Fill in the correct term for each finding:

   Absence of pulse _____

   Apical pulse is greater than the radial pulse _____

   Peripheral vasculature resistance _____

   Respiratory rate below 12 breaths per minute _____

   Irregular pulse rhythm _____

   The difference between diastolic and systolic pressures _____

10. Write out this formula for arterial blood pressure:

$$MAP = CO \times TPR$$

_____

_____

_____

_____

_____

11. Your patient has a screening blood pressure reading of 166/112. What is your recommendation for follow-up?

_____

_____

_____

_____

_____

Self-Assessment Quiz

1. Under which of the following assessments would each patient observation be noted?

_____ Flat affect	A. Stated/apparent age
_____ Tremors and tics	B. Body fat
_____ Diaphoresis	C. Stature
_____ Thin, frail	D. Motor activity
_____ Ataxia	E. Body/breath odor
_____ Slumped	F. Personal hygiene
_____ Long limbs	G. Mood and manner
_____ Disheveled	H. Speech
_____ Slurring	I. Facial expression
_____ Wheezing	J. Distress
_____ Aphasia	

2. Label the following diagram with the pulse sites.

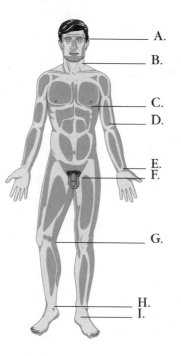

A.
B.
C.
D.
E.
F.
G.
H.
I.

3. List four factors that can affect blood pressure.

(1) _____

(2) _____

(3) _____

(4) _____

4. **True or False?**

    □ **T** □ **F**   Oxygen therapy can affect a patient's oral temperature reading.

    □ **T** □ **F**   The lower edge of the blood pressure cuff should just cover the antecubital fossa.

    □ **T** □ **F**   Hypothermia is a body temperature below 35°C.

    □ **T** □ **F**   Phase III of the Korotkoff sounds is heard as clear, intense tapping.

    □ **T** □ **F**   The resting pulse rate of a 14-year-old approximates that of an adult.

    □ **T** □ **F**   Bradycardia in an adult is a pulse rate below 60; tachycardia is above 110.

    □ **T** □ **F**   The cause of hypertension in 90% of patients who have it is unknown.

    □ **T** □ **F**   An unrecognized auscultatory gap can result in low systolic and high diastolic readings.

    □ **T** □ **F**   A difference of greater than 5 to 10 mm Hg between the blood pressures in both arms is abnormal.

5. Core body temperature can be affected by what physiological variables?

_____

_____

_____

_____

_____

Lab Practice for Skin, Hair, and Nails

Chapter

10

Learning Objectives

1. Conduct a review of systems (ROS) on your lab partner.
2. Demonstrate a physical assessment of the skin, hair, and nails.
3. Describe the characteristics of primary and secondary skin lesions.
4. List the danger signs for cancerous lesions.

Reading Assignment

Prior to beginning this lab assignment, please read Chapter 10, "Skin, Hair, and Nails," in *Health Assessment & Physical Examination* by Mary Ellen Zator Estes, pages 221-264.

Key Terms

Please define the following terms:

Albinism _____

_____

Alopecia_____

_____

Anemia_____

_____

Apocrine Glands _____

_____

Arrector Pili Muscle _____

_____

Carotenemia _____

_____

Cherry Angioma _____

_____

Cyanosis_____

_____

Dehydration _____

_____

Dermis _____

_____

Desquamation _____

_____

Ecchymosis _____

_____

Eccrine Glands _____

_____

Edema _____

_____

Eleidin _____

_____

Epidermis _____

_____

Granulation Tissue _____

_____

Hirsutism _____

_____

Hyperthermia _____

_____

Hypothermia _____

_____

Integumentary System _____

_____

Jaundice _____

_____

Keratosis _____

_____

Lentigo _____

_____

Lesion _____

_____

Lichenification _____

_____

Lunula _____

_____

Mast Cells _____

_____

Matrix _____

_____

Melanocytes _____

_____

Nail Bed _____

_____

Nail Plate _____

_____

Nail Root _____

_____

Nevi _____

_____

Papillary Layer_____

_____

Periungual Tissue _____

_____

Petechiae _____

_____

Polycythemia_____

_____

Pruritus _____

_____

Purpura _____

_____

Rash _____

_____

Reepithelialization _____

_____

Reticular Layer _____

_____

Sebaceous Glands _____

_____

Seborrhea _____

_____

Sebum _____

_____

Spider Angioma_____

_____

Stratum Corneum _____

_____

Stratum Germinativum_____

_____

Stratum Granulosum _____

_____

Stratum Lucidum _____

_____

Stratum Spinosum_____

_____

Subcutaneous Tissue_____

_____

Sweat Glands_____

_____

Terminal Hair _____

_____

Turgor _____

_____

Vellus Hair _____

_____

Venous Star _____

_____

Vitiligo _____

_____

Xerosis_____

_____

Laboratory Activities

1. Label the following items on the drawing:

   Dermis
   Epidermis
   Hair follicle
   Sebaceous (oil) gland
   Subcutaneous tissue
   Sweat gland (eccrine)

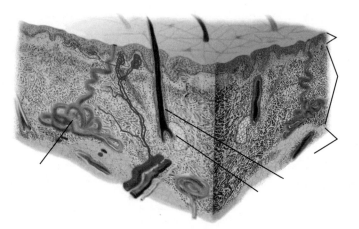

2. How do *apocrine* and *eccrine glands* differ?

_____

_____

_____

_____

_____

3. List five main functions of the skin.

   (1) _____

   (2) _____

   (3) _____

   (4) _____

   (5) _____

4. What is the difference between a *primary* and a *secondary lesion?*

   _____

   _____

   _____

   _____

   _____

5. If your patient had a rash, what questions would you ask for the HPI?

   _____

   _____

   _____

   _____

   _____

6. **ROS (Review of Systems).** Ask your lab partner the following questions:

   _____

   Any history of skin disease or related illness?

   _____

   Unusually dry or moist skin?

   _____

   Any burning, itching, or bruising?

   _____

   Any food, drug, or environmental allergies?

   _____

   Any skin rashes or lesions?

   _____

   Any changes in skin color, pigmentation, or moles?

   _____

   Any changes in or loss of hair?

   _____

On any medications (Rx or OTC)?

Exposure to environmental toxins?   *At work:*

                                             At home:

                                             Hobbies/leisure activities:

*Any significant family hx? (Refer to
pp. 229–230 in your text.)*

How do you care for your skin, hair,   *Skin:*
and nails?
(See p. 232 in your text, Nursing Checklist.)

                                             Hair:

                                             Nails:

7. **Physical Exam.** (*Equipment: Light source, small centimeter ruler, magnifying glass, gloves.*)
   Using your lab partner as a patient, follow the physical assessment guidelines (beginning on
   p. 233 in your text) to complete the following information:

Inspection of the Skin
Color
Bleeding, Ecchymosis, Vascularity
Lesions

Palpation of the Skin
Moisture
Temperature
Texture
Turgor
Edema

Inspection of the Hair
Color
Distribution
Lesions

Palpation of the Hair

Texture _____

Inspection of the Nails

Color _____

Shape and configuration _____

Palpation of the Nails

Texture _____

8. If a lesion is present, what observations should be included in your description?

_____
_____
_____
_____
_____

9. What are the danger signs for potentially cancerous lesions?

_____
_____
_____
_____

10. How do you determine if *edema* is present?

_____
_____
_____
_____

Complete this 4-point grading scale for edema.

_____

+0

_____

+1

_____

+2

_____

+3

_____

+4

_____

11. Explain why *cyanosis* may not be an accurate predictor of oxygen status.

_____

_____

_____

_____

_____

12. What normal variations in color may be noted on a dark-skinned patient?

_____

_____

_____

_____

_____

13. List five changes in the integumentary system associated with aging.

(1) _____

(2) _____

(3) _____

(4) _____

(5) _____

What advice could you give to your elderly patients to help them avoid skin damage?

_____

_____

_____

_____

Self-Assessment Quiz

1. What are some of the characteristics of the skin that you would note on an examination?

_____

_____

_____

_____

2. Which of the following shows an abnormal nail angle?

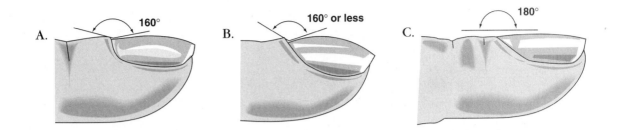

A.   160°

B.   160° or less

C.   180°

3. Identify each of these skin lesions as primary (P) or secondary (S).

_____ Tumor   _____ Papule   _____ Cyst

_____ Keloid   _____ Fissure   _____ Lichenification

_____ Erosion   _____ Ulcer   _____ Pustule

_____ Vesicle   _____ Crust   _____ Scar

4. Match the definition with the correct term.

_____ Localized edema in the epidermis with irregular elevation

_____ Fibrous tissue that replaces dermal tissue after injury

_____ Solid and elevated, deeper than a papule, over 2 cm

_____ Vesicles or bullae filled with pus, less than 0.5 cm diameter

_____ Elevated mass containing serous fluid, less than 0.5 cm

_____ Localized change in skin color, less than 1 cm diameter

_____ Loss of epidermal layers, exposing the dermis

_____ Encapsulated fluid-filled or semi-solid mass in subcutaneous tissue or dermis

A. Vesicle

B. Tumor

C. Freckle

D. Scar

E. Excoriation

F. Wheal

G. Cyst

H. Pustule

5. Name three optimal areas where skin turgor is assessed.

(1) _____

(2) _____

(3) _____

6. Match each lesion with the appropriate diagram.

_____ Linear
_____ Zosteriform
_____ Annular
_____ Confluent

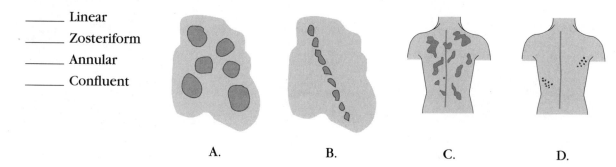

A.   B.   C.   D.

7. **"What's my lesion?"** Read the following descriptions and try to guess what is wrong with these patients.

Patient A has a brownish-pink maculopapular rash that started on the face and neck and now is all over the body. Also has a fever of 101°F, a cough, and Koplik's spots.

Answer: This patient has _____.

Patient B has red, painful vesicles closely grouped together on the trunk, with paresthesia. The lesions follow a dermatome.

Answer: This patient has _____.

Lab Practice for Head and Neck

Learning Objectives

1. Conduct a review of systems (ROS) on your lab partner.
2. Locate anatomical structures of the head and neck.
3. Demonstrate a physical assessment of the head and neck.
4. Differentiate normal and abnormal findings.

Reading Assignment

Prior to beginning this lab assignment, please read Chapter 11, "Head and Neck," in *Health Assessment & Physical Examination* by Mary Ellen Zator Estes, pages 265–284.

Key Terms

Please define the following terms:

Acromegaly _____

_____

Anterior Triangle _____

_____

Atlas _____

_____

Axis _____

_____

Bell's Palsy _____

_____

Bregma _____

_____

Craniosynostosis _____

_____

Craniotabes _____

_____

Down Syndrome _____

_____

Goiter _____

_____

Hydrocephalus _____

_____

Hypertelorism _____

_____

Isthmus (of the Thyroid) _____

_____

Lipoma _____

_____

Posterior Triangle _____

_____

Sutures _____

_____

Torticollis _____

_____

Vertebra Prominens _____

_____

Laboratory Activities

1. Label the following nodes on the drawing:

   Occipital nodes
   Posterior auricular
   Posterior cervical
   Preauricular nodes
   Submandibular nodes
   Submental nodes
   Superficial & deep cervical nodes
   Supraclavicular nodes
   Tonsillar nodes

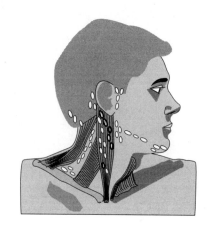

2. Locate each of the following on your lab partner:

Sternocleidomastoid muscle	Mastoid process
Trapezius muscle	Mandible
Temporomandibular joint	Thyroid cartilage
Clavicle	Trachea
Thyroid	External jugular vein

3. Locate the *anterior* and *posterior cervical triangles* on your lab partner. What anatomical features outline each of these areas?

   Anterior: _____

   _____

   Posterior: _____

   _____

4. **ROS (Review of Systems).** Ask your lab partner the following questions:

   _____

   Any history of thyroid, sinus, or related illness?

   _____

   Any surgery on the head or neck?

   _____

   Any history of head injury?

   _____

   Are there any disabilities?

   _____

   Severe or frequent headaches?

   _____

   Any neck pain, tenderness, or swelling?

   _____

   Severe or frequent sore throats?

   _____

   Any change in voice, hoarseness, or difficulty swallowing?

   _____

   Changes in sleep patterns or weight?

   _____

   On any medications (Rx or OTC)?

   _____

   Significant family hx?

   _____

   Use any safety devices for sports or work?

   _____

5. **Physical Exam.** *(Equipment: Stethoscope, cup of water.)* Using your lab partner as a patient, follow the physical assessment guidelines (beginning on p. 272 in your text) to complete the following information:

Inspection of Shape of the Head   _____

Palpation of the Head   _____

Inspection and Palpation of the Scalp   _____

Inspection of the Face
Symmetry   _____
Shape   _____

Palpation and Auscultation of the Mandible   _____

Inspection and Palpation of the Neck
Inspection of the Neck   _____
Palpation of the Neck   _____

Inspection of the Thyroid Gland   _____

Palpation of the Thyroid Gland
Posterior Approach   _____
Anterior Approach   _____

Auscultation of the Thyroid Gland   _____

Inspection of the Lymph Nodes   _____

Palpation of the Lymph Nodes   _____

6. On your lab partner, practice palpating the lymph nodes in a systematic order:

Preauricular
Postauricular
Occipital
Submental
Submandibular
Anterior cervical chain
Posterior cervical chain
Tonsillar
Supraclavicular

(Note: Tonsillar nodes can be palpated after the submandibular nodes.)

7. Examination of the cranial nerves is integrated into your head and neck assessment. How do you evaluate these cranial nerves?

CN #	Name	Method of Evaluation
V		
VII		
XI		

8. What is the technique for assessing the trachea and carotid arteries?

_____

_____

_____

_____

_____

9. List four variations that you might see on the head and neck of an elderly patient.
   (1) _____
   (2) _____
   (3) _____
   (4) _____

Self-Assessment Quiz

1. Draw an outline around the *anterior* and *posterior cervical triangles* on this diagram.

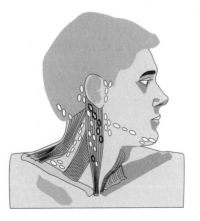

2. Match the following:

_____ Facial asymmetry caused by cranial nerve damage

_____ Caused by premature closure of sutures of the skull

_____ Abnormal enlargement of the skull and face

_____ Associated with hypothyroidism

_____ Autoimmune disorder with increased levels of T_3 and T_4

_____ Sometimes noted in an exam of the TMJ

A. Craniosynostosis

B. Myxedema

C. Bell's palsy

D. Crepitus

E. Acromegaly

F. Graves' disease

3. Label the anatomy in this picture.

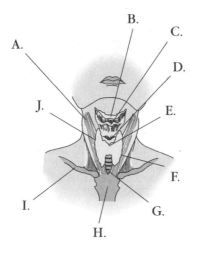

4. **Normal or Abnormal?** You be the judge:

_____ No visible movement of the thyroid while swallowing

_____ Slight lateral deviation of the neck

_____ Small, discrete, movable nodes found on palpation

_____ Solitary nodule in the thyroid tissue

_____ Rubbery, nontender cervical nodes

_____ Inner epicanthal folds on an Asian patient

Lab Practice for Eyes, Ears, Nose, Mouth, and Throat

Chapter 12

Learning Objectives

1. Conduct a review of systems (ROS) on your lab partner.
2. Locate anatomical structures of the eyes, ears, nose, mouth, and throat.
3. Gain competency in using the ophthalmoscope and otoscope.
4. Demonstrate a physical assessment of the eyes, ears, nose, mouth, and throat.

Reading Assignment

Prior to beginning this lab assignment, please read Chapter 12, "Eyes, Ears, Nose, Mouth, and Throat," in *Health Assessment & Physical Examination* by Mary Ellen Zator Estes, pages 285-339.

Key Terms

Please define the following terms:

Accommodation _____

_____

Amblyopia _____

_____

Anisocoria _____

_____

Anterior Chamber_____

_____

Arcus Senilis _____

_____

Auricle _____

_____

Blepharitis _____

_____

Bulbar Conjunctiva_____

_____

Canthus _____

_____

Caruncle _____

_____

Cataract _____

_____

Cerumen _____

_____

Chalazion _____

_____

Chemosis _____

_____

Choroid _____

_____

Ciliary Body _____

_____

Cochlea _____

_____

Coloboma _____

_____

Cones _____

_____

Cornea _____

_____

Dacryoadenitis _____

_____

Dacryocystitis _____

_____

Ectropion (of the Eye) _____

_____

Enophthalmos _____

_____

Entropion _____

_____

Esophoria _____

_____

Esotropia _____

_____

Eustachian Tube _____

_____

Exophoria _____

_____

Exophthalmos _____

_____

Exotropia _____

_____

Fovea Centralis _____

_____

Frenulum (of the Mouth) _____

_____

Glaucoma _____

_____

Hordeolum _____

_____

Hyperopia _____

_____

Hyphema _____

_____

Injection _____

_____

Iris _____

_____

Labyrinth _____

_____

Lacrimal Apparatus _____

_____

Lagophthalmos _____

_____

Lens _____

_____

Limbus _____

_____

Linear Raphe _____

_____

Macula _____

_____

Myopia _____

_____

Nystagmus _____

_____

Optic Disc _____

_____

Ossicles _____

_____

Otitis Media _____

_____

Palpebral Conjunctiva _____

_____

Palpebral Fissure _____

_____

Papilla _____

_____

Paranasal Sinuses _____

_____

Phoria _____

_____

Physiologic Cup _____

_____

Pinguecula _____

_____

Pinna _____

_____

Posterior Chamber _____

_____

Presbycusis _____

_____

Presbyopia _____

_____

Pterygium _____

_____

Ptosis _____

_____

Puncta _____

_____

Pupil _____

_____

Retina _____

_____

Rinne Test _____

_____

Rod _____

_____

Sclera _____

_____

Semicircular Canals _____

_____

Snellen Chart_____

_____

Stensen's Ducts_____

_____

Strabismus _____

_____

Sulcus Terminalis _____

_____

Tarsal Plates_____

_____

Turbinates (or Concha) _____

_____

Uvula _____

_____

Vestibule (of the Ear) _____

_____

Vitreous Humor _____

_____

Weber Test_____

_____

Wharton's Ducts_____

_____

Xanthelasma _____

_____

Laboratory Activities

Eyes

1. How and when would you use the negative and positive diopter settings on the ophthalmo-scope?

_____

_____

_____

_____

_____

2. What anatomical features are you assessing in the retina?

_____

_____

_____

_____

_____

3. **ROS (Review of Systems).** Ask your lab partner the following questions:

_____

Any injury or surgery to the eyes?

_____

Any hx of crossed eyes?

_____

Any change in or loss of vision?

_____

Any eye pain or frequent headaches?

_____

Excessive tearing or dryness?

_____

Use glasses or contact lenses?

_____

Last vision exam/glaucoma testing?

_____

On any medications/eye drops (Rx or OTC)?

_____

Use protective eye wear?

_____

4. **Physical Exam.** *(Equipment: Snellen chart, Rosenbaum near-vision pocket screening card, ophthalmoscope, penlight, cotton-tipped applicator, gloves.)* Using your lab partner as a patient, follow the physical assessment guidelines (beginning on p. 302 in your text) to complete the following information:

Eyes
Visual acuity
    Distance vision   _____
    Near vision   _____
    Color vision   _____
Visual fields   _____

External eye and lacrimal apparatus
   Eyelids   _____
   Lacrimal apparatus   _____
     Inspection   _____
     Palpation   _____
Extraocular muscle function
   Corneal light reflex   _____
   Cover/uncover test   _____
   Cardinal fields of gaze   _____
Anterior segment structures
   Conjunctiva   _____
   Sclera   _____
   Cornea   _____
   Anterior chamber   _____
   Iris   _____
   Pupil   _____
   Lens   _____
Posterior segment structures
   Retinal structures   _____
   Macula   _____

5. How do you test the *corneal light reflex?*

6. What does the *confrontation test* assess?

Which cranial nerve is tested?

7. How would you assess the *direct and consensual light reflex?*

_____

_____

_____

_____

_____

8. What do the *cardinal fields of gaze* assess?

_____

_____

_____

_____

_____

Which cranial nerves are tested? (Give the number and name of each.)

_____

_____

_____

_____

_____

How do you perform this test?

_____

_____

_____

_____

_____

9. Write in the name and number of the cranial nerve that controls each of the eye movements indicated in the following figure.

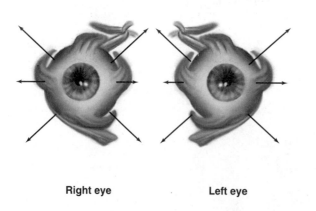

Right eye   **Left eye**

10. Label the following diagram of the retina of the eye with the labels given here:

Artery
Disc margin
Fovea centralis
Macula
Optic disc
Physiologic cup
Vein

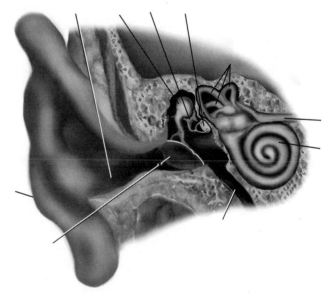

Is this a diagram of the *right* eye or the *left* eye? _____

Ears

11. What are the two pathways for hearing?
    (1) _____
    (2) _____

12. Label the following diagram of a cross-section of the ear.

CN VIII
Cochlea
Eustachian tube
External auditory canal
Helix
Incus
Malleus
Semicircular canals
Stapes
Tympanic membrane

Draw a circle around the *middle ear*.

13. Label the following diagram of the *tympanic membrane*:

Annulus

Handle of the malleus

Junction of incus and stapes

Light reflex

Pars flaccida

Pars tensa

Short process of the malleus

Umbo

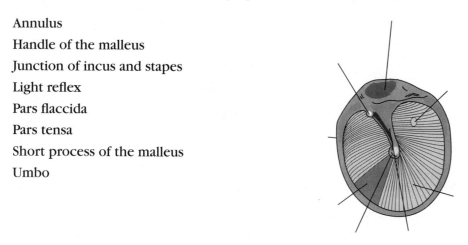

Is this a diagram of the *right* or *left* tympanic membrane? _____

14. Where is the *light reflex* in the right ear? Where is the *light reflex* in the left ear?

_____

_____

_____

_____

_____

15. How do you hold the ear for an otoscopic examination on an adult?

_____

_____

_____

_____

_____

For an examination on a 2-year-old child?

_____

_____

_____

_____

_____

16. **ROS (Review of Systems).** Ask your lab partner the following questions:

_____

Hx of frequent ear infections or tonsilitis?

_____

Any injuries or surgery?

_____

Any earache or ear pain?

_____

Any infection or discharge?

_____

Any ringing, vertigo, hearing loss?

_____

Allergies?

_____

On any medications (Rx or OTC)?

_____

Exposure to excessive noise?

_____

Use of ear protection?

_____

How do you clean your ears?

_____

17. **Physical Exam.** *(Equipment: Otoscope, tuning fork.)* Using your lab partner as a patient, follow the physical assessment guidelines (beginning on p. 319 in your text) to complete the following information:

Ears
Auditory screening
   Voice-whisper test   _____
   Tuning fork tests   _____
      Weber test   _____
      Rinne test   _____
External ear
   Inspection   _____
   Palpation   _____

Otoscopic assessment _____

_____

_____

18. How do you perform the following tests on your lab partner?

Voice-whisper test _____

Weber test _____

Rinne test _____

19. Describe two ways that you can induce movement of the tympanic membrane in your assessment.

_____

_____

_____

_____

_____

Nose, Mouth, and Throat

20. Locate the following anatomical structures on the diagram of the mouth.

Anterior pillar

Gingiva

Palatine tonsil

Papillae

Posterior pharynx

Posterior pillar

Soft palate

Stensen's duct

Uvula

Wharton's duct

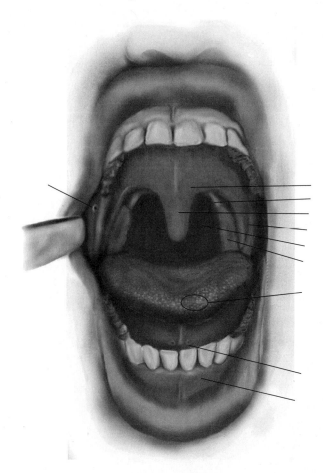

21. How and why would you *transilluminate* the sinuses?

_____

_____

_____

_____

_____

22. Label the following diagram for the *frontal*, *maxillary*, and *ethmoid* sinuses:

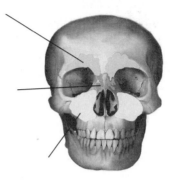

Where are the *sphenoid* sinuses located?

23. **ROS (Review of Systems).** Ask your lab partner the following questions:

_____

Any trauma or injury to the nose, mouth, or throat?

_____

Hx of surgery to nose or throat?

_____

Frequent nosebleeds or nasal discharge?

_____

Frequent colds or allergies?

_____

Any sinus pain or sinusitis?

_____

Any sores in mouth/nose or frequent sore throat?

_____

Any change in sense of smell or taste?

_____

Loose or missing teeth?

_____

On any medications (Rx or OTC)?

_____

Smoking or use of chewing tobacco or alcohol?

_____

Last dental exam and usual dental care?

_____

24. **Physical Exam.** *(Equipment: Otoscope, nasal speculum, penlight, tongue blade, gauze square, gloves.)* Using your lab partner as a patient, follow the physical assessment guidelines (beginning on p. 323 in your text) to complete the following information:

Nose
External inspection   _____
Patency   _____
Internal inspection   _____

Sinuses
Inspection   _____
Palpation and percussion   _____

Mouth and Throat
Mouth
  Breath   _____
  Lips
    Inspection   _____
    Palpation   _____
  Tongue   _____
  Buccal mucosa   _____
  Gums   _____
  Teeth   _____
  Palate   _____
Throat   _____

Special Techniques
Transillumination of the sinuses   _____

25. How do you assess cranial nerves IX, X, and XII?

_____

_____

_____

_____

_____

26. Does your lab partner have tonsils? How would you *grade* them?

_____

_____

_____

_____

_____

What would a grade of *4+* tonsils indicate?

_____

_____

_____

_____

_____

27. Where are the *salivary glands* and their ducts located in the mouth?

Parotid _____

Sublingual _____

Submandibular _____

28. What significant changes occur in the following areas with aging?

Eyes/vision _____

Ears/hearing _____

Mouth/taste _____

What are the three most common visual problems in the elderly population?

(1) _____

(2) _____

(3) _____

Self-Assessment Quiz

1. The area of central vision in the macula is called the _____.

2. Match these terms with the correct description:

_____ Area with a pinpoint reflective center

_____ Tests CN #III, #IV, and #VI

_____ Dilated pupils

_____ Asymmetry indicates deviation in alignment

_____ Can be normal in lateral gaze

_____ Constricted pupils

_____ Tests for peripheral vision

_____ Causes disconjugate vision

_____ Loss of accommodation for near vision

_____ Abnormal retinal structure

A. Strabismus

B. Corneal light reflex

C. Presbyopia

D. Confrontation

E. Neovascularization

F. Macula

G. Cardinal fields of gaze

H. Nystagmus

I. Mydriasis

J. Miosis

3. Lucky you! Your patient has a normal eardrum; please describe it briefly.

_____

_____

_____

_____

_____

4. Sorry, your patient now has a conductive hearing loss on the left side. What results will each of the following tests give?

Weber test: _____

Rinne test: _____

5. **Normal** or **Abnormal?** You be the judge:

_____ Visible peripheral blood vessels on tympanic membrane

_____ Light reflex in right ear at 7:00

_____ Tympanic membrane looks shiny

_____ No lateralization of sound with the Weber test

_____ Small tophus on the auricle

_____ Tympanic membrane moves when patient blows against resistance

6. Here's a challenge: Which of the following are *benign* oral conditions?

Oral hairy leukoplakia	Angular cheilosis	Torus palatinus
Candidiasis	Scrotal tongue	Fibroma
Mandibular tori	Xerostomia	Leukoplakia

Lab Practice for Breasts and Regional Nodes

Learning Objectives

1. Conduct a review of systems (ROS) on your lab partner.
2. Locate anatomical structures of the breasts and regional nodes.
3. Demonstrate a physical assessment of the breasts and regional nodes.
4. Describe a technique for breast self-examination.
5. Identify and describe characteristics of common breast masses.

Reading Assignment

Prior to beginning this lab assignment, please read Chapter 13, "Breasts and Regional Nodes," in *Health Assessment & Physical Examination* by Mary Ellen Zator Estes, pages 341–364.

Key Terms

Please define the following terms:

Acini_____

_____

Alveoli (of the Breast) _____

_____

Areola_____

_____

Augmentation Mammoplasty_____

_____

Axillary Nodes _____

_____

Breasts _____

_____

Colostrum _____

_____

Cooper's Ligaments _____

_____

Ectodermal Galactic Band _____

_____

Granulomatous Reaction (in the Breast) _____

Gynecomastia _____

Lactiferous Ducts _____

Lobes (of the Breast) _____

Lobules (of the Breast) _____

Lymphatic Drainage _____

Mastectomy _____

Milk Line _____

Montgomery's Tubercles _____

Nipple _____

Paget's Disease _____

Peau d'Orange _____

Retromammary Adipose Tissue _____

Supernumerary Nipples _____

Tail of Spence _____

Laboratory Activities

1. Using your lab partner as your patient, locate the following four groups of axillary nodes:

   Central axillary nodes (midaxillary)
   Pectoral (anterior)
   Subscapular (posterior)
   Lateral (brachial)

   Locate the supraclavicular and infraclavicular lymph nodes.

2. Label the following items on the diagram:

Areola
Cooper's ligament
Glandular tissue
Lactiferous duct
Lobes
Nipple
Pectoralis major muscle

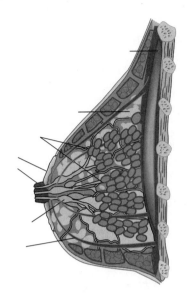

3. At what developmental stage (*sexual maturity rating*) do these changes occur?

_____ Height spurt ends

_____ Menses begins, breast and areola enlarge

_____ Nipple protrudes, areola flush with the breast

_____ Height spurt begins, areola enlarges

_____ Nipple is small, slightly raised

_____ Height spurt peaks

_____ Nipple and breast form a small mound

A. Preadolescent

B. Breast bud

C. Adolescent

D. Late adolescent

E. Adult

4. What are some techniques that can make your patient more comfortable for the breast examination?

_____

_____

_____

_____

_____

5. List at least six risk factors for breast cancer.

(1) _____

(2) _____

(3) _____

(4) _____

(5) _____

(6) _____

6. **ROS (Review of Systems).** Ask your lab partner the following questions:

   _____

   Any trauma, injury, or surgery to the breasts?

   _____

   Changes noted with menstrual cycle?

   _____

   Any pain or tenderness, burning?

   _____

   Any rash, discharge, lumps, dimpling, or swelling?

   _____

   Pregnant or breast feeding? LMP?

   _____

   On any medications (Rx or OTC)?

   _____

   Hx of breast disease (yours or family)?

   _____

   Last breast exam by MD, CNP, or CNM? Mammogram?

   _____

   Performing BSE? Correct technique? How often?

   _____

7. **Physical Exam.** *(Equipment: Towel, drape, small centimeter ruler, teaching aid for breast self-examination.)* Using your lab partner as a patient, follow the physical assessment guidelines (beginning on p. 348 of your text) to complete the following information:

   Inspection
   Color _____
   Vascularity _____
   Thickening/Edema _____
   Size and Symmetry _____
   Contour _____
   Lesions/Masses _____
   Discharge _____

   Palpation
   Supraclavicular lymph nodes _____
   Infraclavicular lymph nodes _____

Breasts (patient sitting)
_____
_____

Axillary lymph nodes
_____

Breasts (patient supine)
_____
_____

8. If you note a mass in your patient's breast, what characteristics do you need to evaluate or describe?

_____
_____
_____
_____
_____
_____

9. If you detect a lump, how can you distinguish between a *cyst* (benign breast disease), a *fibroadenoma*, and *carcinoma*?

Cyst _____
Fibroadenoma _____
Carcinoma _____

10. Using the acronym *BSE*, describe how you would teach the breast self-examination. Include a pattern for systematic palpation and frequency/timing information.

_____
_____
_____
_____
_____
_____

11. Your patient has just turned 40 years old. How often should the following tests be performed?

Mammogram _____
Physical examination _____
Breast self-examination _____

12. List some of the changes that occur in the breast with aging. How would these changes affect the breast examination?

_____
_____
_____
_____
_____

Self-Assessment Quiz

1. You have discovered a lump in your patient's right breast. What characteristics would you include in your description? (List at least five.)

   (1) _____

   (2) _____

   (3) _____

   (4) _____

   (5) _____

2. Which of the following characteristics are more likely to be true for a malignancy than for a cyst or fibroadenoma?

   A. Most common after age 50   E. Well-defined border

   B. Usually mobile   F. Erythema may be present

   C. Usually nontender   G. Associated with retraction and dimpling

   D. Soft to firm consistency   H. Round or ovoid in shape

3. If your patient is a male, can any part of the breast examination be omitted?

   _____

   _____

   _____

   _____

   _____

4. Which of the following are *risk factors* for breast cancer?

   A. Over age 50   E. First baby after 30   I. High-fat diet

   B. Obesity   F. Lives in urban area   J. American

   C. Nulliparous   G. Maternal hx of breast CA   K. Early menarche

   D. Estrogen therapy   H. Higher education   L. European

5. True or False?

   ☐ T ☐ F   Males need a clinical breast examination every one to three years.

   ☐ T ☐ F   Mastectomy patients do not need to perform BSE on the affected side.

   ☐ T ☐ F   Breasts normally feel granular in the elderly patient.

   ☐ T ☐ F   Nipple discharge may be caused by tranquilizers and oral contraceptives.

   ☐ T ☐ F   Supernumerary nipples may be pathologically significant.

   ☐ T ☐ F   Palpable lymph nodes that are more than one centimeter and immobile are usually normal.

6. *Remember these techniques?* What is being performed in each of the following pictures?

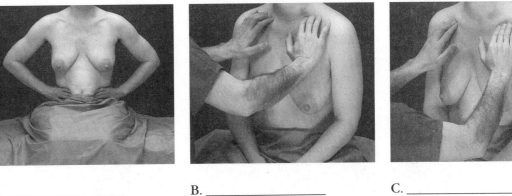

A. _____   B. _____   C. _____

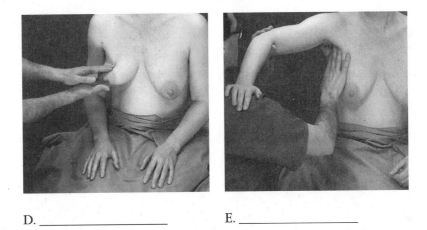

D. _____   E. _____

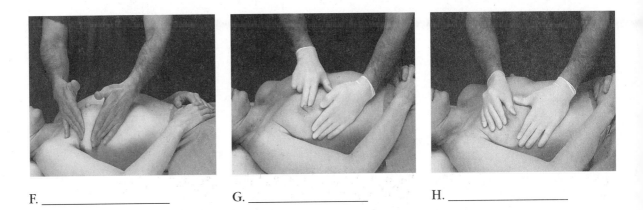

F. _____   G. _____   H. _____

Lab Practice for Thorax and Lungs

Chapter 14

Learning Objectives

1. Conduct a review of systems (ROS) on your lab partner.
2. Locate anatomical landmarks of the thorax and lungs.
3. Differentiate normal and abnormal breath sounds.
4. Demonstrate a physical assessment of the thorax and lungs.

Reading Assignment

Prior to beginning this lab assignment, please read Chapter 14, "Thorax and Lungs," in *Health Assessment & Physical Examination* by Mary Ellen Zator Estes, pages 365–406.

Key Terms

Please define the following terms:

Adventitious Breath Sound _____

_____

Agonal Respirations _____

_____

Air Trapping_____

_____

Alveoli (of the Lung) _____

_____

Angle of Louis (Manubriosternal Junction or Sternal Angle) _____

_____

Anterior Axillary Line _____

_____

Apex (of the Lung) _____

_____

Apnea_____

_____

Apneustic Respirations _____

_____

Ataxic Respirations_____

_____

Barrel Chest _____

_____

Base (of the Lung) _____

Biot's Respirations _____

Bradypnea _____

Bronchial (or Tubular) Breath Sound _____

Bronchophony _____

Bronchovesicular Breath Sound _____

Cheyne-Stokes Respirations _____

Coarse Crackle _____

Costal Angle _____

Costal Margin _____

Cough _____

Crepitus _____

Diaphragmatic Excursion _____

Dyspnea _____

Egophony _____

Eupnea _____

False Ribs _____

Fine Crackle _____

Fissure _____

Floating Ribs _____

Hyperpnea _____

Intercostal Space _____

Interpleural Space _____

Kussmaul's Respirations _____

Kyphosis _____

Manubriosternal Junction _____

Manubrium _____

Mediastinum _____

Midaxillary Line _____

Midclavicular Line _____

Midspinal (or Vertebral) Line _____

Midsternal Line _____

Orthopnea _____

Parietal Pleura _____

Pectus Carinatum _____

Pectus Excavatum _____

Pleura _____

Pleural Friction Fremitus _____

Pleural Friction Rub _____

Posterior Axillary Line _____

_____

Rhonchal Fremitus _____

_____

Scapular Line _____

_____

Scoliosis _____

_____

Sibilant Wheeze _____

_____

Sighing _____

_____

Sonorous Wheeze _____

_____

Sputum _____

_____

Sternal Angle _____

_____

Stridor _____

_____

Suprasternal Notch _____

_____

Tachypnea _____

_____

Tactile (or Vocal) Fremitus _____

_____

Thoracic Expansion _____

_____

True Ribs _____

_____

Tubular Breath Sound _____

_____

Tussive Fremitus _____

_____

Vertebral Line _____

_____

Vertebra Prominens _____

_____

Vertebrosternal (or True) Ribs _____

_____

Vesicular Breath Sound _____

_____

Visceral Pleura_____

_____

Vocal Fremitus _____

_____

Voice Sounds_____

_____

Whispered Pectoriloquy _____

_____

Xiphoid Process _____

_____

Laboratory Activities

1. Label the following items on the drawing:

   Alveoli
   Diaphragm
   Epiglottis
   Esophagus
   Larynx
   Main bronchus
   Mediastinum
   Respiratory bronchiole
   Secondary bronchus
   Trachea

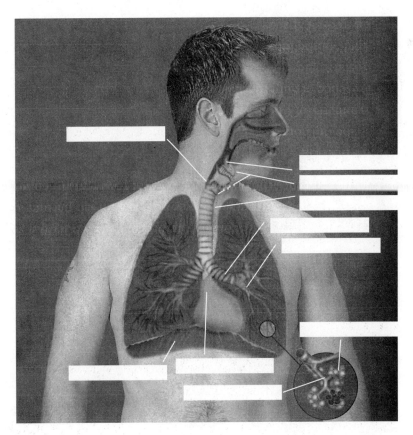

2. Where do the lung apices extend:

   Anteriorly?_____

   Posteriorly? _____

3. At what level is the lower border of the lung:

Anteriorly at the MCL? _____

Posteriorly on inspiration? _____

Posteriorly on expiration? _____

4. Locate the following thoracic anatomical landmarks on your lab partner:

Costal margin	Midaxillary line	Posterior axillary line
Costal angle	Xiphoid process	Vertebral line
Suprasternal notch	Midsternal line	Vertebra prominens
Manubrium of sternum	Midclavicular line	Spinous process of T1
Angle of Louis	Anterior axillary line	

5. What is the normal costal angle?

_____

6. Draw and name the lobes of the lungs and fissures on the diagrams:

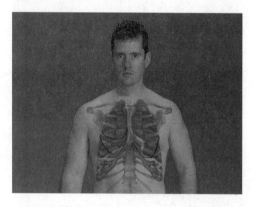

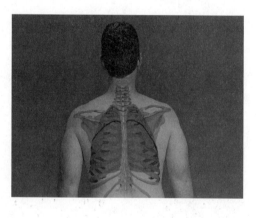

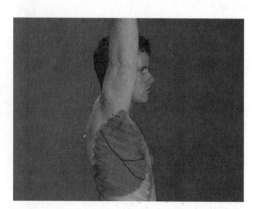

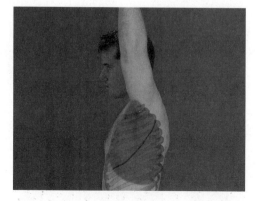

7. Describe the three *normal* breath sounds and determine where they are normally heard.

Breath Sound	Description	Location
Bronchial		
Bronchovesicular		
Vesicular		

8. Which pairs of ribs are each of the following?

False ribs: rib pairs # _____

Floating ribs: rib pairs # _____

Vertebrosternal ribs: rib pairs # _____

9. What is the normal shape of the thorax? How do you determine the ratio of the AP diameter to the transverse diameter?

_____

_____

_____

_____

_____

10. **ROS (Review of Systems).** Ask your lab partner the following questions:

_____

Any hx of lung diseases or surgery?

_____

Any SOB or chest pain?

_____

Any coughing?

_____

Asthma or allergies?

_____

On any medication (Rx or OTC)?

_____

Any sleep problems? (Refer to p. 376 in your text.)

_____

Significant environmental exposure?
(Refer to p. 375 in your text.)

At home?

_____

At work?

_____

Hobbies/leisure?

_____

Any significant family hx?

_____

Last TB test/chest x-ray? Results?

_____

Smoking now or previously?

_____

Recent travel?

_____

Exercise?

_____

Use any safety devices?

_____

Flu vaccine?

_____

11. **Physical Exam.** *(Equipment: Stethoscope, watch with a second hand, centimeter ruler or tape measure, washable marker.)* Using your lab partner as a patient, follow the physical assessment guidelines (beginning on p. 377 in your text) to complete the following information:

Inspection

Shape of Thorax   _____

Symmetry of Chest Wall   _____

Presence of Superficial Veins   _____

Costal Angle   _____

Angle of the Ribs   _____

Intercostal Spaces

Muscles of Respiration

Respirations

    Rate   _____

    Pattern   _____

Depth   _____

Symmetry   _____

Audibility   _____

Patient position   _____

Mode of breathing   _____

Sputum   _____

Palpation

General Palpation

Pulsations   _____

Masses   _____

Thoracic tenderness   _____

Crepitus   _____

Thoracic Expansion   _____

Tactile Fremitus   _____

Tracheal Position   _____

Percussion

General Percussion   _____

Diaphragmatic Excursion   _____

Auscultation

General Auscultation   _____

_____

Breath Sounds   _____

_____

Voice Sounds   _____

_____

Special Techniques

Locating the Site of a Fractured Rib   _____

Forced Expiratory Time   _____

12. How do you assess *diaphragmatic excursion*? What is the normal measurement and at what level?

_____

_____

_____

_____

_____

13. How do you check for each of the following? What will you feel or hear if normal?

Tactile fremitus _____

Bronchophony _____

Egophony _____

Whispered pectoriloquy _____

14. What is the difference between *abnormal* and *adventitious* breath sounds?

_____

_____

_____

_____

_____

Describe the six *adventitious* breath sounds:

	Respiration Phase	Timing	Description	Etiology
Fine crackle				
Coarse crackle				
Sonorous wheeze				
Sibilant wheeze				
Pleural friction rub				
Stridor				

Which two adventitious breath sounds never clear with coughing?

(1) _____

(2) _____

15. Complete the following chart comparing a patient with a pneumothorax to a patient with congestive heart failure (CHF).

	Pneumothorax	**CHF**
Shape of thorax		
Skin color		
Clubbing		
Capillary refill		
Retractions/bulging		
Tactile fremitus		
Tracheal position		
Percussion		
Adventitious sounds		

16. Which changes in the respiratory system of your aging patients make them more susceptible to pneumonia?

What risk factors are probable in a nursing home population?

Self-Assessment Quiz

1. Fill in the blanks:

   The normal breath sound that is auscultated over the periphery of the lung fields is _____
   The three stimuli for breathing are_____
   Nailbed clubbing indicates _____
   Subcutaneous emphysema is also called _____

2. Match each of the following terms with the right definition:

   _____ Muffled, indistinct voice sounds on auscultation   A. Tactile fremitus
   _____ Low-pitched, snoring adventitious sound   B. Pleural effusion
   _____ Adventitious lung sound, coarse and grating
   _____ Abnormal fluid between the layers of the pleura   C. Angle of Louis
   _____ Collapsed, deflated section of alveoli   D. Atelectasis
   _____ Level of the second rib   E. Bronchophony
   _____ Palpable vibration over chest wall when the   F. Friction rub
          patient speaks
                                                                      G. Sonorous wheeze

3. Name each of the following respiratory patterns.

   A. _____   B. _____

   C. _____   D. _____

4. Normal or Abnormal?

   _____ Patient A: Tactile fremitus pronounced at T1 and T2.
   _____ Patient B: Level of diaphragm on inspiration at T10.
   _____ Patient C: Diaphragmatic excursion of 3 cm.
   _____ Patient D: Peripheral breath sounds of high pitch and blowing/hollow
                                    quality.
   _____ Patient E: Barrel chest and kyphosis in an older patient.

5. Match each of the following findings with the probable condition:

_____ Absent breath sounds

_____ Hyperresonance

_____ Absent voice sounds

_____ Rust or blood-tinged sputum

_____ Pleural friction rub

_____ Pink sputum

_____ Fine crackles

_____ Increased tactile fremitus

A. Pneumonia

B. Asthma

C. Pulmonary edema

D. COPD

Lab Practice for Heart and Peripheral Vasculature

Chapter 15

Learning Objectives

1. Identify anatomical structures and landmarks of the heart and peripheral vasculature.
2. Conduct a review of systems (ROS) on your lab partner.
3. Demonstrate a physical assessment of the heart and peripheral vasculature.
4. Differentiate normal and abnormal findings.

Reading Assignment

Prior to beginning this lab assignment, please read Chapter 15, "Heart and Peripheral Vasculature," in *Health Assessment & Physical Examination* by Mary Ellen Zator Estes, pages 407–453.

Key Terms

Please define the following terms:

Afterload _____

_____

Allen Test _____

_____

Angina _____

Apex (of the Heart) _____

_____

Atrial Kick _____

_____

Atrioventricular (A-V) Node _____

_____

Atrioventricular (A-V) Valves _____

_____

Baroreceptors _____

_____

Base (of the Heart) _____

_____

Bruit _____

_____

Cardiomegaly _____

_____

Click _____

_____

Crescendo _____

_____

Decrescendo _____

_____

Diastole _____

_____

Edema _____

_____

Electrodcardiogram (EKG) _____

_____

Gallop _____

_____

Heave _____

_____

Holosystolic _____

_____

Homan's Sign _____

_____

Hyperkinetic _____

_____

Hypokinetic _____

_____

Infarction (Myocardial) _____

_____

Insufficiency _____

_____

Ischemia (Myocardial) _____

_____

Isoelectric Line _____

_____

Lift _____

_____

Orthostatic Hypotension _____

_____

Pallor _____

_____

Palpitation _____

_____

Pansystolic _____

_____

Parietal Pericardium _____

_____

Pericarditis _____

_____

Precordium _____

_____

Preload _____

_____

Pulsus Paradoxus _____

_____

Regurgitation _____

_____

Septum _____

_____

Sinoatrial (S-A) Node _____

_____

Snap _____

_____

Stenosis _____

_____

Syncope _____

_____

Systole _____

_____

Thrill _____

_____

Tilts _____

_____

Visceral Pericardium _____

_____

Laboratory Activities

1. Label the following items on the drawing:

Aortic arch

Diaphragm

Inferior vena cava

Left internal jugular vein

Left lung

Pulmonary trunk

Right internal jugular vein

Right lung

Superior vena cava

Trachea

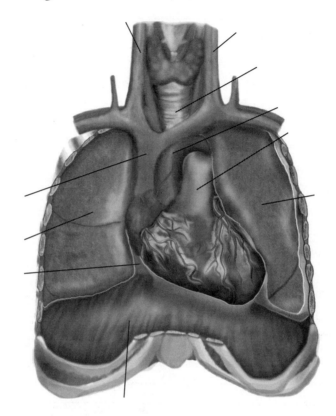

2. Locate the following cardiac landmarks on the diagram:

A   Aortic area

B   Base of the heart

E   Erb's point

M   Mitral area

P   Pulmonic area

T   Tricuspid area

X   Apex of the heart

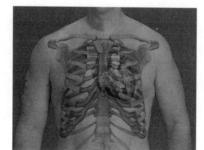

3. Locate the following anatomical landmarks on your lab partner:

Suprasternal notch

Right and left 2nd ICS

Angle of Louis

Cardiac landmarks: aortic, pulmonic, Erb's point, tricuspid, mitral

Peripheral pulses: carotid, brachial, radial, femoral, popliteal, posterior tibial, dorsalis pedis

4. Identify and differentiate S_1 and S_2 and determine where each sound is heard loudest to auscultation.

_____
_____
_____
_____
_____

5. Describe S_3 and S_4. When in the cardiac cycle are these heard?

_____
_____
_____
_____
_____

   What generates these sounds?

_____
_____
_____
_____
_____

6. Explain the physiology of a *split* S_2.

_____
_____
_____
_____
_____

7. Assessment of the *peripheral vasculature* includes:

_____
_____
_____
_____
_____

8. What advice would you give to a patient who is interested in beginning an exercise program?

_____
_____
_____
_____
_____

How would you calculate the *target heart rate* for a 40-year-old patient?

_____

_____

_____

_____

9. How do you inspect for *jugular venous pressure*? What are normal values?

_____

_____

_____

_____

_____

10. What is the difference between a *thrill* and a *heave*?

_____

_____

_____

_____

_____

11. **ROS (Review of Systems).** Ask your lab partner the following questions:

_____

Any hx of heart disease, murmurs, rheumatic fever?

_____

Any bleeding disorders, DM, HTN?

_____

Any hx of chest trauma or surgery?

_____

Any chest pain, SOB, or coughing?

_____

Do you tire easily? Awaken at night to urinate?

_____

Any sores or lesions on your arms or legs?

_____

Any leg cramps, pain, or swelling of feet or legs?

_____

On any medications (Rx or OTC)?

Any exposure to noxious substances at work or home?

Family hx of heart disease?

Any alcohol, tobacco, or drug use?

Do you exercise (activity, duration, and frequency)?

Excessive stress? Often feel angry?

EKG, chest x-ray, serum cholesterol, triglycerides?

12. **Physical Exam.** *(Equipment: Stethoscope, sphygmomanometer, watch with second hand, tape measure.)* Using your lab partner as a patient, follow the physical assessment guidelines (beginning on p. 426 in your text) to complete the following information:

Assessment of the Precordium

Inspection
- Aortic Area
- Pulmonic Area
- Midprecordial Area
- Tricuspid Area
- Mitral Area

Palpation
- Aortic Area
- Pulmonic Area
- Midprecordial Area
- Tricuspid Area
- Mitral Area

Auscultation
- Aortic Area
- Pulmonic Area
- Midprecordial Area
- Tricuspid Area
- Mitral Area

Mitral and Tricuspid Area (S_3)   _____

Mitral and Tricuspid Area (S_4)   _____

Murmurs   _____

Pericardial Friction Rub   _____

Prosthetic Heart Valves   _____

Assessment of the Peripheral Vasculature

Inspection of the Jugular Venous
Pressure   _____

Inspection of the Hepatojugular
Reflux   _____

Palpation and Auscultation of
Arterial Pulses   _____

Inspection and Palpation of Peripheral
Perfusion

Peripheral Pulse   _____

Color   _____

Clubbing   _____

Capillary Refill   _____

Skin Temperature   _____

Edema   _____

Ulcerations   _____

Skin Texture   _____

Hair Distribution   _____

Palpation of the Epitrochlear Node   _____

Special Techniques

Orthostatic Hypotension
Assessment   _____

Assessing for Pulsus Paradoxus   _____

Assessing the Venous System

Homan's Sign   _____

Manual Compression   _____

Retrograde Filling, or
Trendelenburg Test   _____

Assessing the Arterial System

Pallor   _____

Color Return and Venous
Filling Time   _____

Allen Test   _____

Assistive Devices

Artificial Cardiac Pacemakers   _____

Hemodynamic Monitoring   _____

Antiembolic Stockings   _____

Chest Tubes   _____

EKG Monitoring   _____

Intravenous Catheters   _____

Pneumatic Compression Stockings   _____

Pulse Oximetry   _____

13. Document the amplitude of your lab partner's pulses using the stick figure.

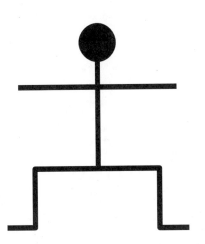

14. Identify the *cardiac risk factors* for your lab partner.

_____

_____

_____

_____

_____

15. Describe the assessment for *orthostatic hypotension*.

_____

_____

_____

_____

_____

16. List the seven characteristics used to describe a *murmur*.

(1) _____

(2) _____

(3) _____

(4) _____

(5) _____

(6) _____

(7) _____

17. Describe how to perform the *Allen Test*.

_____

_____

_____

_____

_____

Why would this technique be performed?

_____

_____

_____

_____

_____

18. Differentiate between venous and arterial ulcerations.

	Arterial Ulcerations	**Venous Ulcerations**
Location		
Characteristics		
Pain		

19. What are the warning signs of imminent cardiovascular problems?

_____

_____

_____

_____

_____

20. What changes occur in the cardiovascular system with aging?

_____

_____

_____

_____

_____

21. What effect can each of the following have on the cardiovascular system of the elderly patient?

COPD _____

Obesity _____

Smoking_____

Osteoporosis _____

Diabetes Mellitus _____

Self-Assessment Quiz

1. What is the normal pathway of blood flow through the heart (including valves)?

   _____

   _____

   _____

   _____

   _____

2. **True or False?**

   □ **T** □ **F** S_1 represents the closing of the aortic and pulmonic (semilunar) valves.

   □ **T** □ **F** S_2 is heard loudest at the base of the heart.

   □ **T** □ **F**   The apex is closer to the 4th/5th ICS; the base is closer to the 2nd ICS.

   □ **T** □ **F**   Erb's Point is auscultated at the 4th ICS left sternal border.

   □ **T** □ **F**   Palpating the carotid arteries simultaneously assists in testing for symmetry.

   □ **T** □ **F**   A thrill is a palpable finding that may be noted with a murmur.

   □ **T** □ **F**   The sound of an S_4 is represented by the word "Kentucky."

   □ **T** □ **F**   A murmur graded V/VI can be heard with the diaphragm held off the chest.

   □ **T** □ **F**   Increased jugular vein distention may be seen in right-sided heart failure.

   □ **T** □ **F**   Blanching in the extremities followed by cyanosis is seen in Raynaud's disease.

3. Identify *systole* and *diastole* on the diagram of the cardiac cycle. Note on the diagram when closure of the *A-V valves* occurs. Draw the *PQRST* wave in relation to the cardiac cycle.

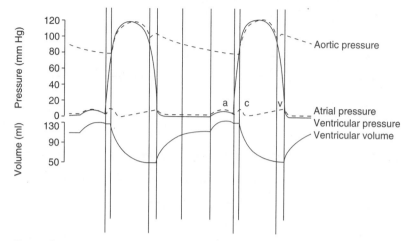

Reproduced with permission from Guyton. A. C. (1995). Textbook of medical physiology (9th ed.). Philadelphia: W. B. Saunders Company.

4. Match the following findings:

_____ Noted at 5th ICS, left midclavicular line

_____ High-pitched, multiphasic, scratchy

_____ Final phase of diastole

_____ Turbulent blood flow

_____ Often associated with an S_3

_____ Noted with palpation

A. Thrill

B. Murmur

C. Mitral valve murmur

D. Heart Failure

E. Pericardial friction rub

F. Atrial kick

5. What are the risk factors for cardiac disease? Circle those that are *fixed*.

_____

_____

_____

_____

_____

6. Match the cardiovascular disorder to its common findings:

_____ Anorexia, fatigue, arthralgia, petechiae

_____ Severe pain, paresthesia, intermittent claudication

_____ SOB, angina, dysrhythmias, nausea, diaphoresis

_____ Diaphoresis, rales, S_3, anxiety, fatigue

_____ Sudden onset, sharp or stabbing pain, anxiety

_____ Dependent edema, hepatomegaly, weight gain

_____ Angina, MI, dysrhythmias, sudden cardiac death

A. Pulmonary embolus

B. CHF (left-sided)

C. CHF (right-sided)

D. Endocarditis

E. Atherosclerosis

F. Myocardial infarction

G. Peripheral vascular disease

Lab Practice for Abdomen

Learning Objectives

1. Conduct a review of systems (ROS) on your lab partner.
2. Locate anatomical structures of the abdomen.
3. Demonstrate a physical assessment of the abdomen.
4. Differentiate normal and abnormal findings.
5. Describe pain assessment techniques.

Reading Assignment

Prior to beginning this lab assignment, please read Chapter 16, "Abdomen," in *Health Assessment & Physical Examination* by Mary Ellen Zator Estes, pages 455-490.

Key Terms

Please define the following terms:

Ascites _____

_____

Ballottement _____

_____

Borborygmi _____

_____

Caput Medusae _____

_____

Cullen's Sign _____

_____

Cutaneous Hypersensitivity _____

_____

Dysphagia _____

_____

Eructation _____

_____

Flatulence _____

_____

Fluid Wave _____

_____

Hematemesis _____

_____

Iliopsoas Muscle Test _____

_____

McBurney's Point _____

_____

Murphy's Sign _____

_____

Obturator Sign _____

_____

Puddle Sign _____

_____

Rebound Tenderness _____

_____

Rovsing's Sign _____

_____

Shifting Dullness _____

_____

Striae _____

_____

Venous Hum _____

_____

Laboratory Activities

1. What is the sequence for examination of the abdomen? Why?

_____

_____

_____

_____

_____

2. Label the following items on the diagram:

Appendix
Ascending colon
Bladder
Descending colon
Gallbladder
Inguinal ligament
Liver
Pancreas
Spleen
Stomach
Transverse colon

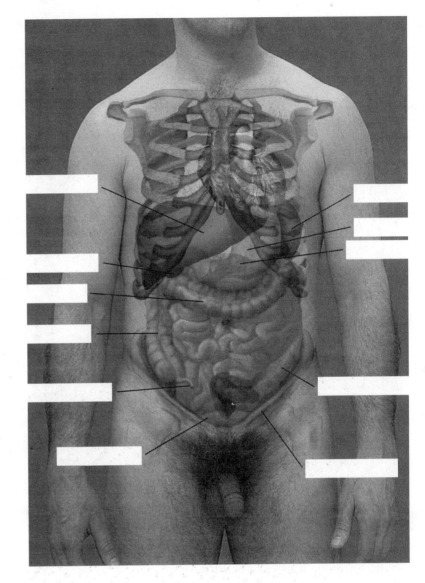

3. List the main function for each of the following:

Stomach _____

Small intestine _____

Large intestine _____

Liver _____

Gallbladder _____

Pancreas _____

Spleen _____

Kidneys _____

4. Locate the following anatomical landmarks on your lab partner:

Xiphoid process   Inguinal ligament   Anterior superior iliac spine

Costal margin   Abdominal midline   Abdominal quadrants

Umbilicus   Symphysis pubis   Rectus abdominis muscle

5. What is the predominate sound heard with percussion of the abdomen? Why?

_____

_____

6. Mark on the diagram where you auscultate for bruits.

    A Abdominal aorta

    R Renal arteries

    I Iliac arteries

    F Femoral arteries

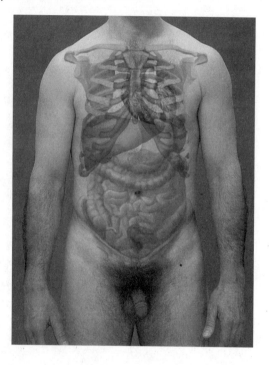

7. How do you handle a ticklish patient during abdominal palpation?

_____

_____

_____

_____

_____

8. **ROS (Review of Systems).** Ask your lab partner the following questions:

_____

Hx of GI disease or surgery?

_____

Any hx of abdominal trauma?

_____

Hx of eating disorders?

Any abdominal pain, nausea, vomiting, or heartburn?

Change in appetite or intolerance to foods?

Diarrhea, distention, or constipation?

Excessive belching or flatulence?

Any difficulty swallowing?

Any dysuria or nocturia?

What is your usual stool pattern (frequency, color, consistency)?

On any medications (Rx or OTC)?

Significant family hx?

LMP? Pregnant?

Use alcohol?

Any recent travel?

What was your previous 24-hour diet hx?

9. **Physical Exam.** *(Equipment: Stethoscope, small centimeter ruler, drape, tangential lighting, marking pencil, sterile safety pin.)* Using your lab partner as a patient, follow the physical assessment guidelines (beginning on p. 467 in your text) to complete the following information:

Inspection

Contour   _____

Symmetry   _____

Rectus Abdominis Muscles   _____

Pigmentation and Color   _____

Scars   _____

Striae   _____

Respiratory Movement   _____

Masses or Nodules   _____

Visible Peristalsis   _____

Pulsation   _____

Umbilicus   _____

Auscultation

Bowel Sounds   _____

Vascular Sounds   _____

Venous Hum   _____

Friction Rubs   _____

Percussion

General Percussion   _____

Liver Span   _____

Liver Descent   _____

Spleen   _____

Stomach   _____

Fist Percussion

   Kidney   _____

   Liver   _____

Bladder   _____

Palpation

Light Palpation   _____

Abdominal Muscle Guarding   _____

Deep Palpation   _____

Liver

   Bimanual Method   _____

   Hook Method   _____

Spleen   _____

Kidneys   _____

Aorta   _____

Bladder   _____

Inguinal Lymph Nodes   _____

Special Techniques

Percussion for Ascites

   Shifting Dullness   _____

   Puddle Sign   _____

Fluid Wave   _____

Murphy's Sign   _____

Rebound Tenderness   _____

Rovsing's Sign   _____

Cutaneous Hypersensitivity   _____

Iliopsoas Muscle Test   _____

Obturator Muscle Test   _____

Ballottement   _____

10. How do you estimate liver span?

_____

_____

_____

_____

_____

   What is the normal liver span for an adult at the MCL?

_____

_____

11. What are the possible causes for abdominal distension?

_____

_____

_____

_____

_____

12. Describe three methods used to assess for ascites.

   (1) _____

   (2) _____

   (3) _____

13. When should you avoid palpation of an area?

_____

_____

_____

_____

_____

14. What are five special techniques that can assess for appendicitis?

Technique   **Method**

(1)

_____

(2)

_____

(3)

_____

(4)

_____

(5)

_____

15. Risk factors for liver cancer include:

_____

_____

_____

_____

16. What changes occur in the abdomen with aging?

_____

_____

_____

_____

17. If your elderly patient complains of a change in bowel habits, what conditions should be considered?

_____

_____

_____

_____

_____

Self-Assessment Quiz

1. The abdomen is located between the _____ and the _____.

2. In which *quadrant* is each of the following located?

_____ Liver	_____ Spleen	A. Right upper
_____ Stomach	_____ Kidneys	B. Right lower
_____ Appendix	_____ Sigmoid colon	C. Left upper
_____ Gallbladder	_____ Descending colon	D. Left lower
_____ Duodenum	_____ Body of the pancreas	

3. Will you use the *diaphragm* or the *bell* of your stethoscope to auscultate these?

_____ Carotid arteries	_____ Femoral artery bruit
_____ Bowel sounds	_____ Voice sounds (lungs)
_____ Thyroid gland	_____ Venous hum
_____ Lungs	_____ Heart

4. **Normal or Abnormal?**

_____ A visible aortic pulsation

_____ Positive borborygmi

_____ Aortic pulsation of 5 cm

_____ Small movable inguinal nodes

_____ Sister Mary Joseph's nodule

_____ Hypoactive bowel sounds

_____ Liver span of 6 cm at the midclavicular line

_____ Negative Rovsing's sign

_____ Small fluid wave

_____ Splenic dullness 9 cm above the costal margin

5. What are the *"Seven Fs"* of abdominal distension?

(1) _____

(2) _____

(3) _____

(4) _____

(5) _____

(6) _____

(7) _____

6. *"Where does it hurt?"*

A. Pain originating in an organ may be experienced in another area. This is called _____.

B. If the patient has abdominal pain, that area should be palpated _____.

C. Before beginning the assessment, ask the patient to _____ to elicit a sharp twinge of pain in the involved area.

D. Lightly palpate the rectus muscles during expiration to determine the presence of

_____.

E. While performing abdominal palpation, observe the patient's face for

_____.

F. *Murphy's sign* is positive in inflammatory processes of the _____.

G. Applying firm pressure to the abdomen and quickly releasing it may produce

_____ in the presence of peritoneal irritation.

H. Pain in the RLQ may indicate _____.

Lab Practice for Musculoskeletal System

Learning Objectives

1. Locate anatomical structures of the musculoskeletal system.
2. Conduct a review of systems (ROS) on your lab partner.
3. Demonstrate a physical assessment of the musculoskeletal system.
4. Describe abnormal gait patterns.

Reading Assignment

Prior to beginning this lab assignment, please read Chapter 17, "Musculoskeletal System," in *Health Assessment & Physical Examination* by Mary Ellen Zator Estes, pages 491–550.

Key Terms

Please define the following terms:

Acromegaly _____

_____

Appendicular Skeleton _____

_____

Atrophy _____

_____

Axial Skeleton _____

_____

Bouchard's Node _____

_____

Bow Legs _____

_____

Bunion _____

_____

Bursae _____

_____

Callus _____

_____

Corn _____

_____

Diaphysis _____

_____

Dislocation _____

_____

Disuse Atrophy _____

_____

Epimysium _____

_____

Epiphyses _____

_____

Ganglion _____

_____

Genu Valgum _____

_____

Genu Varum _____

_____

Goniometer _____

_____

Hallux Valgus _____

_____

Hammer Toe _____

_____

Heberden's Node _____

_____

Hemiparesis _____

_____

Hemiplegia _____

_____

Hypertrophy _____

_____

Hypotonicity _____

_____

Joint _____

_____

Knock Knees _____

_____

Kyphosis _____

_____

Ligament _____

_____

List _____

_____

Lordosis _____

_____

Medullary Cavity _____

_____

Pes Cavus _____

_____

Pes Planus _____

_____

Pes Valgus _____

_____

Pes Varus _____

_____

Polydactyly _____

_____

Scoliosis _____

_____

Spasticity _____

_____

Subluxation _____

_____

Syndactyly _____

_____

Synovial Effusion _____

_____

Tendons _____

_____

Thenar Eminence _____

_____

Laboratory Activities

1. Label each of the bones on this diagram:

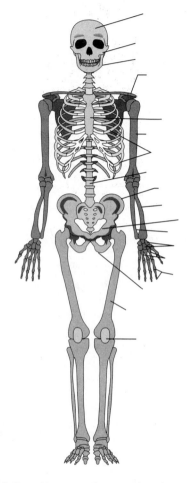

2. Label the following muscles on the diagram:

   Biceps

   Deltoid

   External oblique

   Iliopsoas

   Masseter

   Pectoralis major

   Quadriceps femoris

   Rectus abdominis

   Sartorius

   Serratus anterior

   Sternocleidomastoid

   Temporalis

   Tibialis anterior

   Triceps

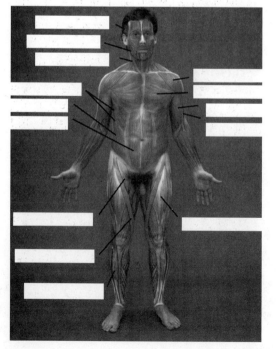

3. Locate the following major bone and muscle structures on your lab partner:

Humerus	Patella	Metatarsals	Vertebral column	Biceps
Ulna	Femur	Metacarpals	Sternum	Triceps
Radius	Fibula	Clavicle	Trapezius	Quadriceps
Carpals	Tibia	Maxilla	Gluteus maximus	Deltoid
Tarsals	Mandible	Phalanges	Rectus abdominis	

4. What patients require a complete musculoskeletal assessment?

_____

_____

_____

_____

_____

What does a screening, or musculoskeletal *mini-assessment*, include?

_____

_____

_____

_____

_____

5. Have your lab partner perform these skeletal muscle movements:

Flexion	Internal rotation	Elevation	Inversion
Extension	External rotation	Depression	Eversion
Abduction	Pronation	Protraction	Dorsiflexion
Adduction	Supination	Retraction	Plantar flexion
Rotation	Circumduction	Hyperextension	Lateral bending

6. Describe these *synovial* joints and give an example of each:

Joint	Description	Example
Hinge		
Pivot		
Saddle		
Condyloid		

Ball and socket

Gliding

7. Describe two techniques used in assessing for *carpal tunnel syndrome*.

What types of activities might lead to this injury?

8. Describe six *range of motion* movements for the shoulder.
    (1) _____
    (2) _____
    (3) _____
    (4) _____
    (5) _____
    (6) _____

9. **ROS (Review of Systems).** Ask your lab partner the following questions:

Hx of broken bones, sprains, dislocations, or other trauma?

Any bone or joint deformity?

Any joint stiffness, swelling, redness, or pain?

Frequent or severe back pain?

Any loss of mobility, strength, or endurance?

Can you perform all daily activities (lifting, walking, pushing, pulling, etc.)?

_____

On any medication (Rx or OTC)?

_____

Any strenuous activities at work, home, or sports?

_____

Repetitive motion activities for work or hobbies?

_____

Any significant family hx?

_____

Use alcohol or tobacco?

_____

Do you exercise (type, duration, frequency)?

_____

Use safety devices at work or for sports?

_____

10. **Physical Exam.** *(Equipment: Goniometer, cloth measuring tape, sphygmomanometer and blood pressure cuff, washable marker.)* Using your lab partner as a patient, follow the physical assessment guidelines (beginning on p. 501 in your text) to complete the following information:

    General Assessment
    Overall Appearance   _____
    Posture   _____
    Gait and Mobility   _____
                                _____
                                _____

    Inspection
    Muscle Size and Shape   _____
    Joint Contour and Periarticular
    Tissue   _____

    Palpation
    Muscle Tone   _____
    Joints   _____

    Range of Motion   _____
                                _____

Muscle Strength

_____

_____

Examination of Joints

Temporomandibular Joint

Cervical Spine

Shoulders

Elbows

Wrists and Hands

Hips

Knees

Ankles and Feet

Spine

Special Techniques

Measuring Limb Circumference

Using a Goniometer

Assessing for Chvostek's Sign

Drop Arm Test

Assessing for Trousseau's Sign

Assessing Grip Strength Using a
Blood Pressure Cuff

Assessing for Tinel's Sign

Assessing for Phalen's Sign

Trendelenburg Test

Measuring Limb Length

Patrick's Test

Assessing for Bulge Sign

Patellar Ballottement

Assessing for Apley's Sign

Assessing for McMurray's Sign

Drawer Test

Lachman's Test

Assessing Status of Distal Limbs
and Digits

Thompson Test

Assessing for Scoliosis

Straight Leg Raising Test
(Lasègue's Test)

Milgram Test

Assistive Devices

Crutches _____

Cane _____

Walker _____

Brace, Splint, Immobilizer _____

Cast _____

Skin Traction _____

Skeletal Traction _____

External Fixation _____

11. Describe the body mechanics of an erect posture and a normal gait.

_____

_____

_____

_____

_____

_____

12. How can you differentiate between *osteoarthritis* and *rheumatoid arthritis*?

_____

_____

_____

_____

_____

_____

13. What is the significance of the notation S3/T2/L3?

_____

_____

_____

_____

_____

_____

14. What are the differences among *scoliosis*, *kyphosis*, and *lordosis*?

_____

_____

_____

_____

_____

_____

Which is often seen in the pregnant patient? _____

Which is found with osteoporosis? _____

Which is seen in elderly patients? _____

How do you assess for scoliosis?

_____

_____

_____

_____

_____

15. What special techniques can be used to examine the knee?

Technique	Method	Etiology
Bulge sign		
Patellar ballottement		
Apley's sign		
McMurray's sign		
Drawer test		
Lachman's test		

16. What are the "Five Ps" of *neurovascular deterioration*?
    (1) _____
    (2) _____
    (3) _____
    (4) _____
    (5) _____

17. What changes might you see in the musculoskeletal system of an elderly female patient?

_____

_____

_____

_____

_____

18. How do age-related changes affect the ability of the elderly patient to perform ADLs?

_____

_____

_____

_____

_____

19. List signs that may indicate elder abuse or neglect.

_____

_____

_____

_____

_____

Self-Assessment Quiz

1. Match the following special techniques:

_____ Is positive in neuroexcitability	A. Drawer test
_____ Detects large effusions in the knee	B. Lachman's test
_____ Assesses the integrity of the meniscus	C. Trousseau's sign
_____ Is positive with a rupture of the Achilles tendon	D. Bulge sign
_____ Tests for small effusions in the knee	E. Apley's sign
_____ Detects loose or movable objects in the knee	F. Thompson test
_____ Checks the stability of cruciate ligaments	G. Patellar ballottement
_____ Assesses stability of the anterior cruciate ligament	H. McMurray's sign

2. Since your patient has "complete ROM against gravity with moderate resistance," you grade this muscle strength as a _____ on a scale of _____.

3. **True or False?**

   ☐ **T** ☐ **F**   Osteoarthritis may cause joints to appear hot, tender, and painful, with possible deformities.

   ☐ **T** ☐ **F**   Bouchard and Heberden's nodes are findings in rheumatoid arthritis.

   ☐ **T** ☐ **F**   You ask your patient (nicely) to do a shoulder shrug to test CN XII.

   ☐ **T** ☐ **F**   Rotator cuff damage is demonstrated in the drop arm test.

   ☐ **T** ☐ **F**   A positive Trendelenburg test indicates hip dislocation.

   ☐ **T** ☐ **F**   Osteoporosis produces uneven shoulders and hip levels that can be detected by having the patient bend over.

4. Match each of the following findings:

_____ Slow, writhing, twisting movement

_____ Pes planus

_____ Visible twitching of muscle fibers

_____ Genu valgum

_____ Enlargement of skull, hands, feet, and long bones

_____ Sudden, rapid muscle spasms in upper body

_____ Genu varum

_____ Hallux valgus

A. Knock knees

B. Bow legs

C. Flat foot

D. Bunion

E. Tic

F. Fasciculation

G. Athetosis

H. Acromegaly

5. **True or False?**

☐ **T** ☐ **F**   *Festinating* is seen in Parkinson's disease.

☐ **T** ☐ **F**   An *apraxic* gait is slow and shuffling.

☐ **T** ☐ **F**   *Cerebellar ataxia* causes the patient to stagger and sway.

☐ **T** ☐ **F**   With muscular dystrophy or hip dysplasia, a *"waddling"* gait may be seen.

☐ **T** ☐ **F**   Causes of abnormal gait include muscle weakness, joint deterioration, paralysis, lack of coordination and balance, fatigue, and pain.

6. Label each of these abnormalities of the spine:

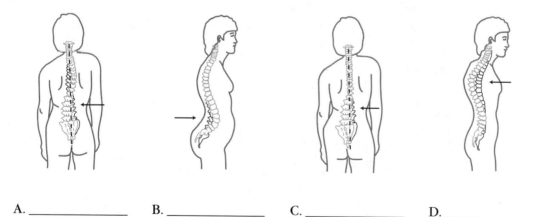

A. _____   B. _____   C. _____   D. _____

7. And your Final Jeopardy answer is: "This test will assess for a herniated lumbar disc."

For the Grand Prize, the question is: _____?

Lab Practice for Mental Status and Neurological Techniques

Chapter 18

Learning Objectives

1. Identify anatomical structures in the neurological system.
2. Conduct a review of systems (ROS) on your lab partner.
3. Demonstrate a mental status examination and physical assessment of the neurological system.
4. Differentiate normal and abnormal findings.

Reading Assignment

Prior to beginning this lab assignment, please read Chapter 18, "Mental Status and Neurological Techniques," in *Health Assessment & Physical Examination* by Mary Ellen Zator Estes, pages 551–604.

Key Terms

Please define the following terms:

Ageusia _____

_____

Agnosia _____

_____

Agraphia _____

_____

Alexia _____

_____

Analgesia _____

_____

Anesthesia _____

_____

Anosmia _____

_____

Aphasia _____

_____

Aphonia _____

_____

Apraxia _____

_____

Astereognosis _____

_____

Bell's Palsy _____

_____

Clonus _____

_____

Confabulation _____

_____

Constructional Apraxia _____

_____

Decerebrate Rigidity _____

_____

Decorticate Rigidity _____

_____

Dermatome _____

_____

Dysarthria _____

_____

Dyscalculia _____

_____

Dysdiadochokinesia _____

_____

Dysesthesia _____

_____

Dysmetria _____

_____

Dysphonia _____

_____

Dyssynergy _____

_____

Echolalia _____

_____

Glasgow Coma Scale _____

_____

Graphanesthesia _____

_____

Graphesthesia _____

_____

Hypalgesia _____

_____

Hyperalgesia _____

_____

Hyperesthesia _____

_____

Hypesthesia _____

_____

Hypoesthesia _____

_____

Hypogeusia _____

_____

Paresthesia _____

_____

Perseveration _____

_____

Proprioception _____

_____

Seizure _____

_____

Stereognosis _____

_____

Syncope _____

_____

Vertigo _____

_____

Word Blindness _____

_____

Laboratory Activities

1. Label the following items on the drawing:

   Broca's area
   Cerebellum
   Diencephalon
   Frontal lobe
   Medulla oblongata
   Midbrain
   Occipital lobe
   Parietal lobe
   Pons
   Spinal cord
   Temporal lobe
   Wernicke's area

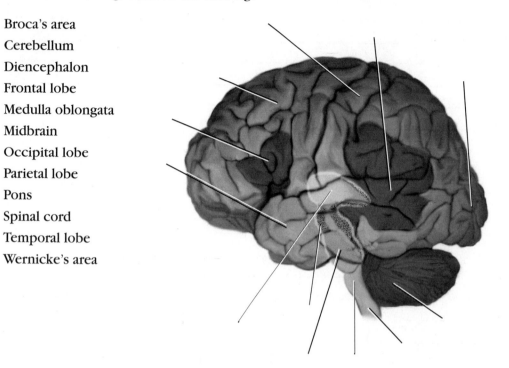

2. How do the *sympathetic* and *parasympathetic* nervous systems differ?

   _____
   _____
   _____
   _____
   _____

3. Name the three categories of reflexes and give three examples of each:

   Category   **Examples**
   _____   _____
                                          _____
                                          _____
   _____   _____
                                          _____
                                          _____
   _____   _____
                                          _____
   _____   _____

4. What items are included in a *mental status* exam?

_____

_____

_____

_____

_____

5. What is one technique (sensory or motor) for assessing each of the *cranial nerves*?

CN #	Name	Assessment Technique
I		
II		
III		
IV		
V		
VI		
VII		
VIII		
IX		
X		
XI		
XII		

6. How could you assess *coordination* in the *upper* extremities?

_____

_____

_____

_____

_____

How could you assess coordination in the *lower* extremities?

_____

_____

_____

_____

7. **ROS (Review of Systems).** Ask your lab partner the following questions:

_____

Any head or spinal cord injuries?

_____

Any hx of stroke, meningitis, alcoholism, or hypertension?

_____

Hx of congenital defects?

_____

Any hx of psychiatric illness or treatment for an emotional disturbance?

_____

Hx of communicable disease such as polio, AIDS, syphilis, rickettsial infections?

_____

Any fainting, dizziness, loss of coordination, or weakness?

_____

Any numbness, tingling, or tremors?

_____

Any changes in visual acuity or visual fields?

_____

Having problems with recent or remote memory loss?

_____

Any difficulty with speaking or swallowing?

_____

Are you experiencing chronic or unusual stress?

_____

On any medication (Rx or OTC)?

_____

Use alcohol, tobacco, or street drugs?

_____

Any environmental or occupational hazards?

_____

Family hx of neurological or psychiatric disorders?

_____

Use safety devices where appropriate?

_____

8. **Physical Exam.** *(Equipment: Reflex hammer, tuning fork, tongue blade, penlight, cotton-tipped applicators, cotton ball, sterile safety pin, familiar small objects (coins, key, paperclip), vials of odorous materials (coffee, etc.), vials of hot and cold water, vials with solutions for tasting, Snellen chart, pupil gauge.)* Using your lab partner as a patient, follow the physical assessment guidelines (beginning on p. 565 in your text) to complete the following information:

Mental Status Assessment

Physical Appearance and Behavior

   Posture and Movements _____

   Dress, Grooming, and

      Personal Hygiene _____

   Facial Expression _____

   Affect _____

Communication _____

Level of Consciousness _____

Cognitive Abilities and Mentation

   Attention _____

   Memory _____

   Judgment _____

   Insight _____

   Spatial Perception _____

   Calculation _____

   Abstract Reasoning _____

   Thought Process and

      Content _____

Sensory Assessment

Exteroceptive Sensation

   Light Touch _____

   Superficial Pain _____

   Temperature _____

Proprioceptive Sensation

   Motion and Position _____

   Vibration Sense _____

Cortical Sensation

   Stereognosis _____

   Graphesthesia _____

   Two-Point Discrimination _____

   Extinction _____

Cranial Nerves Assessment

Olfactory Nerve (CN I) _____

Optic Nerve (CN II)

   Visual Acuity _____

   Visual Fields _____

   Funduscopic Examination _____

Oculomotor Nerve (CN III)

   Cardinal Fields of Gaze _____

   Eyelid Elevation _____

   Pupil Reactions _____

Trochlear Nerve (CN IV)

   Cardinal Fields of Gaze _____

Trigeminal Nerve (CN V)

   Motor Component _____

   Sensory Component _____

Abducens Nerve (CN VI)

   Cardinal Fields of Gaze _____

Facial Nerve (CN VII)

   Motor Component _____

   Sensory Component _____

Acoustic Nerve (CN VIII)

   Cochlear Division

      Hearing _____

      Weber Test _____

      Rinne Test _____

   Vestibular Division _____

Glossopharyngeal Nerve (CN IX) _____

Vagus Nerve (CN X) _____

Spinal Accessory Nerve (CN XI) _____

Hypoglossal Nerve (CN XII) _____

Motor System Assessment

Muscle Size _____

Muscle Tone _____

Muscle Strength _____

Involuntary Movements _____

Pronator Drift _____

Cerebellar Function

Coordination _____

Station _____

Gait _____

Reflexes

Deep Tendon Reflexes

Biceps _____

Brachioradialis _____

Triceps _____

Patellar _____

Achilles _____

Superficial Reflexes

Abdominal _____

Plantar _____

Cremasteric _____

Bulbocavernosus _____

Pathological Reflexes

Grasp _____

Snout _____

Glabellar _____

Sucking _____

Clonus _____

Babinski _____

Hoffmann's Sign _____

Trömner's Sign _____

Chaddock's Sign _____

Oppenheim's Sign _____

Gordon's Sign _____

Special Techniques

Doll's Eyes Phenomenon _____

Romberg's Test _____

Meningeal Irritation

   Nuchal Rigidity _____

   Kernig's Sign _____

   Brudzinski's Sign _____

9. Document your lab partner's *deep tonal reflexes* (DTRs) and *superficial reflexes* on the stick figure.

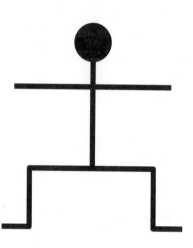

10. Complete the grading scale for DTRs.

_____

1+

_____

2+

_____

3+

_____

4+

_____

11. Describe the following techniques for assessment of *meningeal irritation*.

Kernig's sign _____

Nuchal rigidity _____

Brudzinski's sign _____

12. How would you score your lab partner's *LOC* using the *Glasgow Coma Scale*?

_____

_____

_____

_____

_____

13. If your lab partner displays a positive *Romberg's test*, what is happening?

_____

_____

_____

_____

_____

How would your findings compare for a patient with cerebellar disease and a patient with posterior column disease?

_____

_____

_____

_____

_____

_____

14. Differentiate *decerebrate* and *decorticate rigidity*.

_____

_____

_____

_____

_____

15. What neurological changes in the elderly patient could contribute to the onset of depression?

_____

_____

_____

_____

_____

16. What cognitive and sensory changes might interfere with the elderly patient's ability to perform activities of daily living?

_____

_____

_____

_____

_____

17. How might the characteristics of a patient in Stage I of *Alzheimer's disease* be confused with normal changes often associated with the aging process?

_____

_____

_____

_____

_____

Self-Assessment Quiz

1. Each of the following patients shows an abnormal finding in which cognitive function?

   A. Attention   E. Spatial Perception
   B. Memory   F. Calculation
   C. Judgment   G. Abstract Reasoning
   D. Insight   H. Thought Process/Content

   _____ Patient 1: Can't explain the meaning of "A squeaky wheel gets the grease"

   _____ Patient 2: Gives an inappropriate answer to "What would you do if you saw a house burning?"

   _____ Patient 3: Can't recall a list of three items after a five-minute conversation

   _____ Patient 4: Displays agnosia and constructional apraxia

   _____ Patient 5: Uses confabulation when answering

   _____ Patient 6: Is euphoric

   _____ Patient 7: Is unable to repeat a given sequence of numbers

2. Which deep tendon reflexes are shown here?

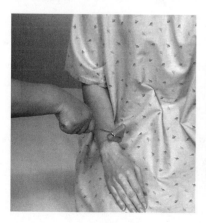 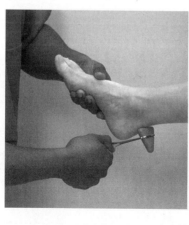 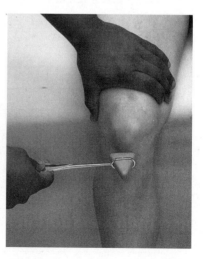

A. _____   B. _____   C. _____

3. **True or False?**

   ☐ **T** ☐ **F** *Broca's area* is responsible for auditory comprehension.

   ☐ **T** ☐ **F** The *posterior column* carries vibration and fine-touch sensations.

   ☐ **T** ☐ **F** Reflexes are classified as muscle stretch, superficial, or pathological.

   ☐ **T** ☐ **F** *Parasympathetic* responses do not affect pupil size or urine output.

   ☐ **T** ☐ **F** The *GCS* assesses patients on eye opening and reflexes.

   ☐ **T** ☐ **F** *Dyssynergy* and *dysmetria* are abnormal findings in cerebellar function.

   ☐ **T** ☐ **F** The presence of normal *Doll's eyes phenomenon* is noted in patients with a low brain stem lesion.

4. **"Oh, what nerve . . . "** (cranial nerve, that is)?

   Affects strength of trapezius muscles: CN #_____

   Allows patient to produce guttural sounds: CN #_____

   Ageusia and Bell's palsy are abnormal findings: CN #_____

   20/25 OD, 20/20 OS, 20/20 OU: CN #_____

5. And now for the $64,000 question: What techniques assess for meningeal irritation?

   _____

Lab Practice for Female Genitalia

Learning Objectives

1. Locate anatomical structures of the female genitalia.
2. Conduct a review of systems (ROS) on a female lab partner or patient.
3. Demonstrate a physical assessment of the female genitalia.
4. Differentiate normal and abnormal findings.

Reading Assignment

Prior to beginning this lab assignment, please read Chapter 19, "Female Genitalia," in *Health Assessment & Physical Examination* by Mary Ellen Zator Estes, pages 605-639.

Key Terms

Please define the following terms:

Adnexa _____

_____

Amenorrhea _____

_____

Anal Orifice _____

_____

Bartholin's Glands (Greater Vestibular Glands) _____

_____

Cervix _____

_____

Chadwick's Sign _____

_____

Chancre _____

_____

Chandelier's Sign _____

_____

Clitoris _____

_____

Cystocele _____

_____

Cystourethrocele _____

_____

Dysmenorrhea _____

_____

Dyspareunia _____

_____

Ectropion (or Eversion, of the Cervix) _____

_____

Escutcheon _____

_____

Fallopian Tubes _____

_____

Fourchette _____

_____

Fornices _____

_____

Frenulum (of the Female Genitalia) _____

_____

Fundus _____

_____

Hymen _____

_____

Isthmus (of the Uterus) _____

_____

Labia Majora _____

_____

Labia Minora _____

_____

Menarche _____

_____

Menopause _____

_____

Menorrhagia _____

_____

Mons Pubis _____

_____

Nabothian Cysts _____

_____

Nulliparous _____

_____

Oogenesis _____
_____

Ovaries_____
_____

Parous _____
_____

Perineum _____
_____

Rectocele_____
_____

Rectouterine Pouch _____
_____

Rectovaginal Septum _____
_____

Skene's Glands (Paraurethral Glands) _____
_____

Spinnbarkeit _____
_____

Squamocolumnar Junction _____
_____

Uterus _____
_____

Vagina _____
_____

Vaginal Introitus _____
_____

Vestibule _____
_____

Laboratory Activities

1. Note the location of the following anatomical landmarks:

Bartholin's gland
Clitoris
Fourchette
Hymen
Labia majora
Labia minora
Mons pubis
Perineum
Skene's glands
Urethral meatus
Vaginal introitus

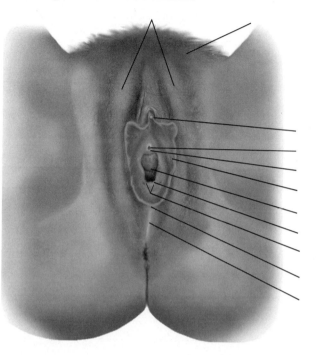

2. Label the following items on the drawing:

Cervix
External os
Fallopian tube
Internal os
Ovary
Posterior fornix
Rectum
Sacrum
Symphysis pubis
Urinary bladder
Uterus
Vagina

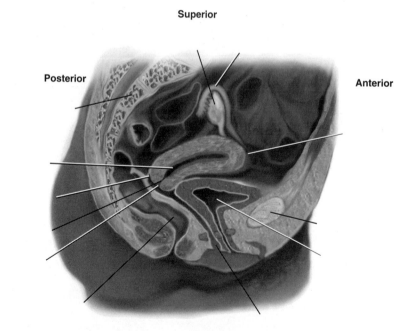

3. What strategies may help your patient feel more comfortable prior to, during, and after the genital assessment?

_____

_____

_____

_____

_____

4. What *cyclic changes* are occurring in the menstrual cycle at the time of ovulation?

_____

_____

_____

_____

_____

What happens to the basal body temperature at ovulation?

_____

_____

_____

_____

_____

How does cervical mucus change at ovulation?

_____

_____

_____

_____

_____

5. What characteristics will you note on inspection of the cervix and cervical os?

_____

_____

_____

_____

_____

6. Describe normal palpation findings of the ovaries.

_____

_____

_____

_____

_____

7. **ROS (Review of Systems).** Ask your lab partner the following questions:

_____

Any hx of disease or surgery to the genitalia?

_____

Hx of vaginal infections, STDs, infertility, CA?

_____

Any pelvic pain, vaginal discharge or bleeding?

_____

Age of menarche? LMP?

_____

Duration and frequency of menses, amount of flow?

_____

Any PMS, spotting between menses, or dysmenorrhea?

_____

Any previous or current pregnancy?

_____

Any symptoms of menopause?

_____

In a satisfactory sexual relationship? Any concerns?

_____

On any medication (Rx or OTC)?

_____

Significant family hx?

_____

Previous Pap smear results?

_____

Method of birth control?

_____

Protection against STDs?

_____

8. **Physical Exam.** *(Equipment: Vaginal specula, gooseneck lamp, drape, examination table with stirrups, warm water, water-soluble lubricant, gloves.)* Using your lab partner or a female patient, follow the physical assessment guidelines (beginning on p. 616 in your text) to complete the following information:

Inspection of the External Genitalia

Pubic Hair Distribution   _____

Presence of Parasites   _____

Skin Color and Condition

   Mons Pubis and Vulva   _____

   Clitoris   _____

   Urethral Meatus   _____

   Vaginal Introitus   _____

   Perineum and Anus   _____

Palpation of the External Genitalia

Labia   _____

Urethral Meatus and Skene's

   Glands   _____

Vaginal Introitus   _____

Perineum   _____

Speculum Examination of the Internal Genitalia

Cervix

   Color   _____

   Position   _____

   Size   _____

   Surface Characteristics   _____

   Discharge   _____

   Shape of the Cervical Os   _____

Collecting Specimens for Cytological Smears and Cultures

Pap Smear   _____

Endocervical Smear   _____

Cervical Smear   _____

Vaginal Pool Smear   _____

Gonococcal Culture Specimen   _____

Saline Mount or "Wet Prep"   _____

KOH Prep   _____

Five Percent Acetic Acid Wash   _____

Anal Culture   _____

Inspection of the Vaginal Wall _____

Bimanual Examination

Vagina _____

Cervix _____

Fornices _____

Uterus _____

Adnexa _____

Rectovaginal Examination _____

9. Compare the following abnormal findings for *vaginal discharge*:

	Color	Odor	Consistency	Cervix
Nonspecific vaginitis				
Trichomonas				
Candida				
Gonococcal				

10. What are the signs of *sexual abuse* in the female patient?

_____

_____

_____

_____

11. The warning signs of an ectopic pregnancy include:

_____

_____

_____

_____

12. What are the risk factors for cancer of the female genitalia?

Cervical cancer _____

_____

Endometrial cancer _____

_____

Ovarian cancer _____

_____

What special population is at risk for *vaginal cancer?*

_____

_____

_____

_____

_____

13. What parts of the female examination are omitted for a patient with a hysterectomy?

_____

_____

_____

_____

_____

14. Describe normal findings on examination of the ovaries, uterus, cervix, and vaginal walls in the elderly patient.

_____

_____

_____

_____

_____

15. What normal changes in the aging process may lead to each of the following problems?

Vaginal infections _____

Uterine prolapse _____

Dyspareunia _____

Self-Assessment Quiz

1. The *Pap smear* consists of three specimens, including:

(1) _____

(2) _____

(3) _____

2. **True or False?**

☐ **T** ☐ **F**   The cervical os in a nulliparous woman is a small horizontal slit.

☐ **T** ☐ **F**   A Thayer-Martin culture plate is used to detect *chlamydia trachomatis*.

☐ **T** ☐ **F**   The cervix is pale after menopause and blue during pregnancy.

☐ **T** ☐ **F**   Swelling or redness around the urethral meatus may indicate a urinary tract infection.

☐ **T** ☐ **F**   Smoking is a risk factor for cervical cancer.

☐ **T** ☐ **F**   *Strawberry spots* on the surface of the cervix may indicate a gonococcal infection.

☐ **T** ☐ **F**   The uterus in the nongravid patient is pear-shaped.

☐ **T** ☐ **F**   Bulging on the posterior vaginal wall may indicate a cystocele.

3. In what order would these assessments be performed?

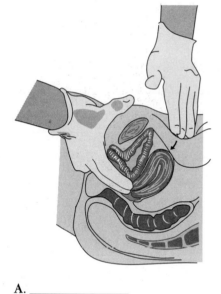

A. _____

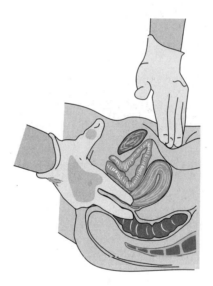

B. _____

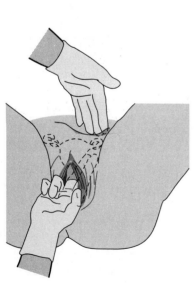

C. _____

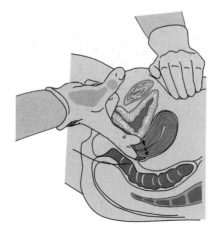

D. _____

4. What's wrong with each of these patients?

Patient A is complaining of a discharge that is grayish yellow and has a fishy odor; the discharge appears purulent.

This patient may have _____.

Patient B has a white discharge with a consistency of cottage cheese. There is no odor, but the vaginal mucosa and vulva appear reddened.

This patient may have _____.

Patient C has several white, dry, painless growths that have a narrow base on the vulva.

This patient may have _____.

Patient D has small, shallow, red vesicles that fuse together into a large ulcer on the vulva, with pain and itching.

This patient may have _____.

5. The presence of what finding on palpation of the cervix may indicate *PID*?

_____

_____

_____

_____

_____

Lab Practice for Male Genitalia

Learning Objectives

1. Identify anatomical structures of the male genitalia.
2. Conduct a review of systems (ROS) on a male lab partner or patient.
3. Demonstrate a physical assessment of the male genitalia.
4. Differentiate normal and abnormal findings.

Reading Assignment

Prior to beginning this lab assignment, please read Chapter Chapter 20, "Male Genitalia," in *Health Assessment & Physical Examination* by Mary Ellen Zator Estes, pages 641–665.

Key Terms

Please define the following terms:

Alopecia _____

_____

Bulbourethral Glands _____

_____

Chancre _____

_____

Chancroid _____

_____

Condyloma Acuminatum _____

_____

Cryptorchidism _____

_____

Direct Inguinal Hernia _____

_____

Ductus (Vas) Deferens _____

_____

Ejaculatory Ducts _____

_____

Epididymis _____

_____

Epispadias _____

_____

Femoral Hernia _____

_____

Glans Penis _____

_____

Hydrocele _____

_____

Hypospadias _____

_____

Impotence _____

_____

Indirect Inguinal Hernia _____

_____

Microphallus _____

_____

Orchitis _____

_____

Paraphimosis _____

_____

Penis _____

_____

Phimosis _____

_____

Prepuce _____

_____

Priapism _____

_____

Scrotum _____

_____

Seminal Vesicles _____

_____

Smegma _____

_____

Spermatic Cord _____

_____

Spermatocele _____

_____

Spermatogenesis _____

_____

Testes_____

_____

Urethra_____

_____

Varicocele _____

_____

Laboratory Activities

1. Label the following items on the drawing:

   Bladder
   Cowper's gland
   Ductus deferens
   Epididymis
   Glans penis
   Prostate gland
   Scrotum
   Seminal vesicle
   Testis
   Ureter
   Urethra

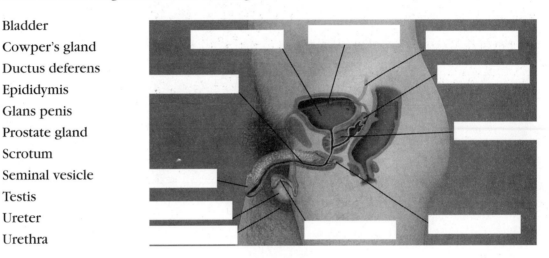

2. What strategies may be helpful when examining the male genitalia?

   _____

   _____

   _____

   _____

   _____

3. Describe normal palpation findings of the testicles and epididymis.

   _____

   _____

   _____

   _____

   _____

   _____

4. What are the warning signs of a hernia?

   _____

   _____

   _____

   _____

   _____

How would you palpate the inguinal area for hernias?

_____

_____

_____

_____

_____

5. **ROS (Review of Systems).** Ask your lab partner or male patient the following questions:

_____

Any hx of disease, surgery, or trauma to the genitalia?

_____

Any urethral discharge, dysuria, or pain?

_____

Any lumps, hernias, scrotal or prostate enlargement?

_____

Sexual dysfunction?

_____

Hx of DM, HTN, CAD, CA?

_____

Any growths on penis?

_____

On any medications (Rx or OTC)?

_____

Any exposure to STDs?

_____

Significant family hx?

_____

Use alcohol, tobacco, or drugs?

_____

Exposure to radiation?

_____

Use condoms? Supportive devices for sports?

_____

Perform TSE? How often?

_____

6. **Physical Exam.** *(Equipment: Stethoscope, penlight, sterile cotton swabs, gloves.)* Using your lab partner or a male patient, follow the physical assessment guidelines (beginning on p. 650 in your text) to complete the following information:

Inspection

Hair Distribution _____

Penis _____

Scrotum _____

Urethral Meatus _____

Inguinal Area _____

Palpation

Penis _____

Urethral Meatus _____

Scrotum _____

Inguinal Area _____

Auscultation

Scrotum _____

Special Techniques

Androscopy _____

Urethral Culture _____

Transillumination of the Scrotum _____

7. Describe each of these *sexually transmitted diseases*.

STD	Lesion	Causative Agent
Syphilis		
Genital warts		
Genital herpes simplex		

8. How would you teach *testicular self-examination* (TSE) to a male patient?

_____

_____

_____

_____

_____

During what part of your examination should TSE be taught?

_____

_____

_____

_____

9. Compare *indirect*, *direct*, and *femoral* hernias.

Hernia	Occurrence	Location	Cause
Indirect Inguinal			
Direct Inguinal			
Femoral			

How would you reduce a direct inguinal hernia?

_____

_____

_____

_____

_____

10. If your patient has a penile discharge, what characteristics would you note?

_____

_____

_____

_____

11. What changes occur in the male genitalia with aging?

_____

_____

_____

_____

12. Aging may affect sexual function by:

_____

_____

_____

_____

_____

Self-Assessment Quiz

1. What are the warning signs of *testicular cancer*?

_____

_____

_____

_____

_____

2. Match the following terms and descriptions:

_____ Spontaneous descent after age one is unusual	A. Testicular torsion
_____ Can be caused by mumps, varicella	B. Testicular tumor
_____ May accompany CHF and renal failure	C. Epididymitis
_____ Feels like a "bag of worms" to palpation	D. Orchitis
_____ Usually caused by bacterial pathogens from urethra	E. Cryptorchidism
_____ A surgical emergency	F. Scrotal edema
_____ Nodular, associated with painless swelling	G. Varicocele

3. Auscultation of a scrotal mass is performed to determine _____.

4. True or False?

☐ **T** ☐ **F** Hypospadias occurs when the urethral meatus opens dorsally on the glans.

☐ **T** ☐ **F** A chancroid is the lesion of primary syphilis and is highly infectious.

☐ **T** ☐ **F** A male patient may be unaware of an HPV infection for months or years.

☐ **T** ☐ **F** Small (1 cm) mobile lymph nodes in the inguinal area are normal.

☐ **T** ☐ **F** Oval swelling at the symphysis pubis is noted with a femoral hernia.

☐ **T** ☐ **F** The left testicle is normally lower in the scrotal sac than the right.

☐ **T** ☐ **F** Transillumination of the scrotum may occur in spermatocele and hernia.

5. Warning signs of *STDs* in the male patient include:

_____

_____

_____

_____

_____

Lab Practice for Anus, Rectum, and Prostate

Learning Objectives

1. Locate anatomical structures of the rectum and prostate gland.
2. Conduct a review of systems (ROS) on your lab partner.
3. Demonstrate a physical assessment of the rectum and prostate gland.
4. Differentiate normal and abnormal findings.

Reading Assignment

Prior to beginning this lab assignment, please read Chapter 21, "Anus, Rectum, and Prostate," in *Health Assessment & Physical Examination* by Mary Ellen Zator Estes, pages 667–685.

Key Terms

Please define the following terms:

Anal Canal _____

_____

Anal Columns _____

_____

Anal Fissure _____

_____

Anal Incontinence _____

_____

Anal Orifice _____

_____

Anal Sinuses _____

_____

Anal Valves _____

_____

Anoderm _____

_____

Anorectal Abscess _____

_____

Anorectal Fistula _____

_____

Anorectum _____

_____

Defecation _____

_____

Hemorrhoids _____

_____

Melena _____

_____

Prostate _____

_____

Rectal Prolapse _____

_____

Rectum _____

_____

Steatorrhea _____

_____

Laboratory Activities

1. Label the following anatomical structures:

   Anal canal
   Anorectal junction
   Bladder
   Bulbourethral (Cowpcr's) gland
   Prostate gland
   Rectum

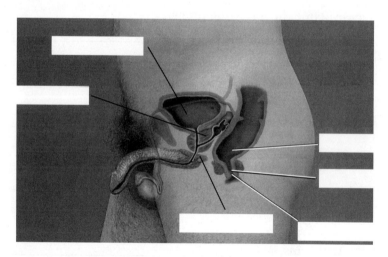

2. What measures can increase your patient's comfort with the rectal/prostate exam?

   _____

   _____

   _____

   _____

   _____

3. **ROS (Review of Systems).** Ask your lab partner the following questions:

Hx of bowel or prostate disease or surgery?

Hx of STDs or rectal trauma?

Hemorrhoids, itching, masses, polyps?

Constipation, diarrhea, or incontinence?

Use alcohol, tobacco, drugs?

Significant family hx?

Any pain or discharge of blood from the rectum?

Any change in weight or appetite?

Any changes in stool?

On any medications (Rx or OTC)?

Excessive stress?

Excessive fats, cured/smoked meats, or insufficient fiber in your diet?

Exercise?

Use condoms during intercourse?

Ever had a colonoscopy?

4. **Physical Exam.** (*Equipment: Water-soluble lubricant, hemoccult cards, lamp, gloves.*) Using your lab partner or a patient, follow the physical assessment guidelines (beginning on p. 674 in your text) to complete the following information:

Inspection

Perineum and Sacrococcygeal
   Area
      _____

Anal Mucosa
      _____
      _____

Palpation

Anus and Rectum
      _____
      _____

Prostate
      _____
      _____

5. What are some common causes of *rectal bleeding*?

_____
_____
_____
_____
_____

6. Risk factors for *rectal cancer* include:

_____
_____
_____
_____
_____

7. What assessment findings may lead you to suspect *rectal abuse*?

_____
_____
_____
_____
_____

8. A 45-year-old patient who is a sexually active homosexual is at risk for what anal, rectal, or prostate problems?

_____
_____
_____
_____
_____

9. What are the causes for each of the following problems in the aging population?

Urinary obstruction _____

_____

Fecal incontinence _____

_____

Rectal prolapse _____

_____

Constipation _____

_____

UTIs _____

_____

10. What teaching might you include to help your elderly patients alleviate some of these symptoms?

_____

_____

_____

_____

_____

Self-Assessment Quiz

1. What are the risk factors for *prostate* cancer?

_____

_____

_____

_____

_____

2. Match the terms with the right description:

_____ Related to aging and the presence of testosterone   A. Hemorrhoids

_____ Results from upper gastrointestinal bleeding   B. Anal fissure

_____ Noted in malabsorption syndrome   C. Rectal prolapse

_____ May result from heavy lifting, childbirth, or straining   D. Melena

_____ Firm, hard, or indurated nodules may be noted   E. Steatorrhea

_____ Appears as pinkish red "doughnut" at anal orifice   F. Prostate cancer

_____ Often seen in Crohn's disease   G. Benign prostatic
                                                                        hypertrophy

3. **True or False?**

☐ T ☐ F   There is a strong association between HSV-2 and anal carcinoma.

☐ T ☐ F   Prostatic abscesses are associated with diabetes mellitus.

☐ T ☐ F   Rectal polyps occur frequently in the general population of the United States.

☐ T ☐ F   Bacterial prostatitis is usually caused by *Escherichia coli.*

☐ T ☐ F   The larger the prostate gland palpated, the greater the symptoms experienced.

☐ T ☐ F   Mucoid or creamy exudate from the rectum is a finding in gonococcal proctitis.

4. The *primary* risk factor for *rectal cancer* is _____.

5. Name the assessment technique that is demonstrated in each of these pictures.

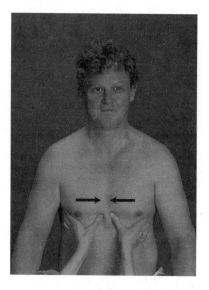

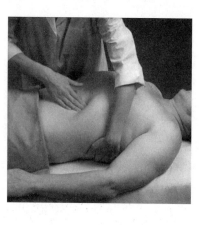

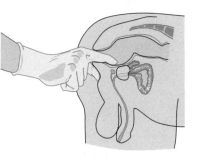

A. _____   B. _____   C. _____

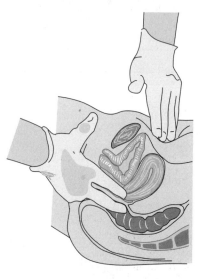

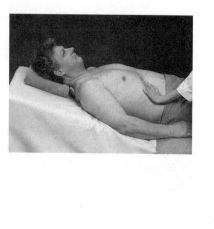

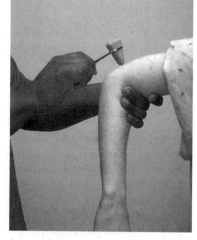

D. _____   E. _____   F. _____

Lab Practice for Pregnant Patient

![black bar]

Learning Objectives

1. Collect information for an obstetrical history.
2. Describe alterations in the physiological system of the pregnant patient.
3. Demonstrate a physical assessment of the pregnant patient.
4. Demonstrate Leopold's maneuver and fundal height measurement.

Reading Assignment

Prior to beginning this lab assignment, please read Chapter 22, "Pregnant Patient," in *Health Assessment & Physical Examination* by Mary Ellen Zator Estes, pages 689–714.

Key Terms

Please define the following terms:

Braxton Hicks Contractions _____

_____

Chloasma _____

_____

Colostrum _____

_____

Diastasis Recti _____

_____

Eclampsia _____

_____

Ectopic Pregnancy _____

_____

Ectropion (or Eversion, of the Cervix) _____

_____

False Labor _____

_____

Fetoscope _____

_____

Friability _____

_____

Glycosuria _____

_____

HELLP Syndrome _____

_____

Hyperemesis Gravidarum _____

_____

Lightening _____

_____

Linea Nigra _____

_____

Macrosomia _____

_____

Melasma _____

_____

Nevi _____

_____

Nocturia _____

_____

Proteinuria _____

_____

Prurigo _____

_____

Ptyalism _____

_____

Quickening _____

_____

Striae Gravidarum _____

_____

Laboratory Activities

1. Write out *Naegele's rule* for determining the delivery date based on the LMP.

_____

_____

_____

_____

_____

Using Naegele's rule, what is the *EDD* (or *EDC*) for each of these patients?

	LMP	**EDD/EDC**
Patient A	February 3	
Patient B	June 15	
Patient C	December 30	

2. What does each of the following sets of abbreviations mean?

G: 4   P: 2   A: 2   LC: 2 _____

G: 2   P: 0   A: 2   LC: 0 _____

G: 3   P: 2   A: 0   LC: 2 _____

3. What are the danger signs of pregnancy?

_____

_____

_____

_____

_____

4. Note some of the normal and abnormal findings in the following physiological systems for the pregnant patient:

System	Normal Changes	Abnormal Findings
Skin and hair		
Head and neck		
Eyes, ears, nose, mouth, and throat		
Breasts		
Thorax and lungs		
Heart and peripheral vasculature		

Abdomen

_____

Urinary system

_____

Musculoskeletal system

_____

Neurological system

_____

Hematological system

_____

Endocrine system

_____

Female genitalia

_____

5. **ROS (Review of Systems).** Ask your lab partner (or pregnant patient) the following questions regarding her present and previous obstetric history:

_____

When was the LMP?

_____

Hx since LMP (fever, rashes, disease or toxic exposure, abnormal bleeding, nausea and vomiting)

_____

Signs and symptoms of pregnancy?

_____

Used fertility drugs?

_____

EDD/EDC

_____

Genetic predispositions (yours or FOB)?

_____

Gravidity, parity, full-term, preterm, number of living children, spontaneous and therapeutic abortions?

_____

Dates of deliveries?

Vaginal or Cesarean section?

Any complications with prior pregnancies?

Length of labor, medications or anesthesia used?

Infant weight, sex, Apgar score, type of feeding?

Any postpartum or breastfeeding complications?

Hx of uterine or abdominal injury or surgery?

On any medications (Rx or OTC)?

Hx of asthma, diabetes, cardiac or renal disease?

Exposure to communicable disease? Rubella immune?

Any alcohol, tobacco, or drug use?

6. **Physical Exam** *(Equipment: Stethoscope, Doppler/fetoscope, centimeter tape measure, watch with a second hand.)* Using your lab partner or a pregnant patient, follow the physical assessment guidelines (beginning on p. 705 in your text) to complete the following information:

Fundal Height

Fetal Heart Rate

Leopold's Maneuver
First maneuver
Second maneuver
Third maneuver
Fourth maneuver

7. Your patient is 36 weeks pregnant with her first child. What recommendations will you have for each of the following items?

Frequency of prenatal checkups: _____

_____

Lab work: _____

_____

Teaching needs: _____

_____

8. A uterine size that is larger than expected (according to LMP) may indicate:

_____

_____

_____

_____

_____

A uterine size smaller than expected may indicate:

_____

_____

_____

_____

_____

9. Your pregnant diabetic patient is at increased risk for what complications?

_____

_____

_____

_____

_____

10. How would you determine if your patient has PIH versus chronic hypertension?

_____

_____

_____

_____

_____

Self-Assessment Quiz

1. Which of these lab results of the pregnant patient needs follow-up?

   Mild glycosuria   HCT 34%

   HGB 14%   Glucose screen 150 mg/dl post glucola

   Rh negative   Trace of proteinuria

2. What do you know about these important *first* events?

   A. Quickening is typically *first* noted by the pregnant woman at _____ weeks.

   B. If a pregnancy is "at-risk," fetal kick counts should *first* be done at _____ weeks.

   C. A Doppler can *first* be used to hear FHTs at _____ weeks.

   D. The *first* Leopold's maneuver determines _____.

   E. A woman pregnant for the *first* time will be a "gravida _____ para _____."

   F. If a pregnant patient has edema, hypertension, and proteinuria, the caregiver should *first*
      suspect _____.

3. Please match the following terms and definitions for the pregnant patient.

   _____ Most common cause of proteinuria   A. Chloasma

   _____ Cervical softening   B. Eclampsia

   _____ Occurs with descent of presenting fetal part into the pelvis   C. Chadwick's sign

   _____ Softening of the uterine isthmus   D. PIH

   _____ Most common cause of seizures   E. Goodell's sign

   _____ Bluish hue to the cervix   F. Abruptio placenta

   _____ Blotchy, irregular pigmentation   G. Diastasis recti

   _____ Separation of abdominal muscle   H. Lightening

   _____ One of the most common causes of abdominal pain   I. Hegar's sign

4. The following drawings show a nurse palpating the abdomen to determine positioning of the fetus. What is the name of this technique?

_____

Identify the proper sequence:

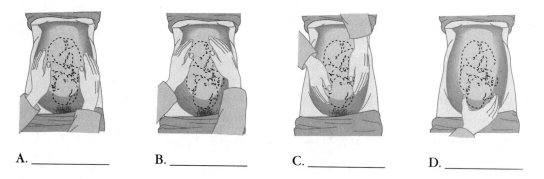

A. _____   B. _____   C. _____   D. _____

5. **Normal or Abnormal?**

_____ A fundus measured at 2 cm above the umbilicus at 22 weeks

_____ Nitrates in the urine

_____ FHTs showing tachycardia at 26 weeks

_____ A drop in fundal height at 40 weeks

_____ Hyperreflexia

_____ A white, milky cervical discharge

Lab Practice for
Pediatric Patient

![black bar]

Learning Objectives

1. Compare physiological variations between pediatric and adult patients.
2. Conduct a review of systems (ROS) on a pediatric patient.
3. Demonstrate a physical assessment of a pediatric patient.
4. Differentiate normal and abnormal findings.
5. Describe strategies that facilitate assessment on an infant or child.

Reading Assignment

Prior to beginning this lab assignment, please read Chapter 23, "Pediatric Patient," in *Health Assessment & Physical Examination* by Mary Ellen Zator Estes, pages 715-769.

Key Terms

Please define the following terms:

Acrocyanosis _____

_____

Anencephaly _____

_____

Apgar Scoring _____

_____

Attention Deficit Hyperactivity Disorder (ADHD)_____

_____

Brushfield's Spots _____

_____

Caput Succedaneum_____

_____

Cephalhematoma _____

_____

Club Foot_____

_____

Cradle Cap_____

_____

Craniosynostosis _____

_____

Craniotabes _____

_____

Cryptorchidism _____

_____

Developmental Dislocation of the Hip _____

_____

Diaphragmatic Hernia _____

_____

Epstein's Pearls _____

_____

Harlequin Color Change _____

_____

Hydrocephalus _____

_____

Intussusception _____

_____

Lanugo _____

_____

Meconium _____

_____

Metatarsus Varus _____

_____

Microcephaly _____

_____

Milia _____

_____

Molding _____

_____

Mongolian Spots _____

_____

Physiological Weight Loss _____

_____

Stork Bites _____

_____

Telangiectatic Nevi _____

_____

Vernix Caseosa _____

_____

Laboratory Activities

1. List the structural and physiological variations in each of the following systems in a child:

System	Variations
Vital signs	
Skin and hair	
Head	
Eyes and Ears	
Nose, mouth, throat	
Breasts	
Thorax and lungs	
Heart and peripheral vasculature	
Abdomen	
Musculoskeletal	
Neurological	
Female genitalia	
Male genitalia	

2. What is the purpose of the *Denver II* tool?

_____

_____

_____

_____

_____

How is the Denver II administered?

_____

_____

_____

_____

_____

3. According to the Denver II tool, at what age are 90% of children able to:

Drink from a cup?_____

Copy a circle? _____

Imitate speech sounds? _____

Roll over?_____

4. How do you perform *Apgar scoring* of a newborn?

_____

_____

_____

_____

_____

What are possible causes of a low Apgar score?

_____

_____

_____

_____

_____

5. Until what age should each of the following be assessed?

Ortolani's maneuver_____

Head circumference_____

Chest circumference _____

6. What general approaches to the pediatric assessment may help your patient be more comfortable and cooperative?

For the infant?

_____

_____

_____

_____

_____

For the toddler/preschooler?

_____

_____

_____

_____

_____

For the older child?

_____

_____

_____

_____

_____

7. Describe the method for eliciting each of the following reflexes in the newborn.

Reflex	Method	Normal Response
Rooting		
Sucking		
Palmar grasp		
Tonic neck		
Stepping		
Plantar grasp		

Babinski's

_____

Moro

_____

Placing

_____

Gallant

_____

Landau

_____

8. Describe three methods for holding an infant and a child for an otoscopic examination.

   (1) _____

   (2) _____

   (3) _____

9. **ROS (Review of Systems).** Ask a pediatric patient or caregiver the following questions:

   (Source and reliability of information?)

   _____

   When mother's prenatal care began?

   _____

   Full-term birth? Preterm?

   _____

   Any complications of pregnancy, labor, or birth?

   _____

   Any hospitalizations or ER visits?

   _____

   Frequent injuries or accidents?

   _____

   Any exposure to measles, mumps, rubella, pertussis, or chicken pox?

   _____

   Current on immunizations?

   _____

   Any significant family hx, including SIDS, congenital defects, or mental retardation?

   _____

Any change in sleep patterns?

_____

Any regression to outgrown behaviors noted?

_____

Any unusual physical complaints?

_____

Frequent episodes of illness?

_____

Sleeping patterns?

_____

Any concerns or problems with current eating habits?

_____

Activities the child enjoys?

_____

How child expresses anger or copes with stress?

_____

In daycare?

_____

Measures taken to childproof the home?

_____

10. **Physical Exam.** *(Equipment: Scale, appropriate-sized blood pressure cuff, Snellen E chart, Allen cards, otoscope speculum (2.5 or 4.0 mm), pediatric stethoscope, growth chart, small bell, brightly colored object, Denver II materials.)* On a pediatric patient, follow the physical assessment guidelines (beginning on p. 732 in your text) to complete the following information:

Developmental Assessment
Denver II   _____

Physical Growth
Weight   _____
Length/Height   _____
Head Circumference   _____
Chest Circumference   _____

Physical Assessment
Apgar Scoring   _____

Head

   Inspection

      Head Control   _____

   Palpation

      Anterior Fontanel   _____

      Posterior Fontanel   _____

      Suture Lines   _____

      Surface Characteristics   _____

Eyes

   Vision Screening

      Allen Test   _____

Musculoskeletal System

   Inspection

      Tibiofemoral Bones   _____

   Palpation

      Feet (Metatarsus Varus)   _____

      Hip and Femur (Ortolani
      Maneuver)   _____

Neurological System

   Rooting   _____

   Sucking   _____

   Palmar Grasp   _____

   Tonic Neck   _____

   Stepping   _____

   Plantar Grasp   _____

   Babinski   _____

   Moro (Startle)   _____

   Gallant   _____

   Placing   _____

   Landau   _____

Special Techniques

Transillumination of the Skull   _____

Assessing for Choanal Atresia   _____

Assessing for Coarctation of the Aorta   _____

11. How can you assess the cranial nerves on a toddler or preschooler?

_____

_____

_____

_____

_____

12. What behavioral changes might be noted in an infant with *congestive heart failure*?

_____

_____

_____

_____

_____

What respiratory signs might be exhibited?

_____

_____

_____

_____

_____

13. List possible signs that might be noted on the skin of a *physically abused* child.

_____

_____

_____

_____

_____

14. What are possible signs of *sexual abuse* in children?

_____

_____

_____

_____

_____

15. What are some safety tips that you might include in your teaching for the parents of an infant?

_____

_____

_____

_____

_____

16. Which immunizations will you administer to your one-year-old patient?

_____

_____

_____

_____

_____

Self-Assessment Quiz

1. According to averages, a baby who weighs 8 pounds and is 20 inches in length at birth would be expected:

   At six months: to weigh _____, with a length of _____
   At one year: to weigh _____, with a length of _____

2. Match the following findings on the newborn:

   _____ Changes from pale to ruddy color at midline
   _____ Premature ossification of suture lines
   _____ Seborrheic dermatitis
   _____ Localized, subcutaneous swelling over a cranial bone
   _____ Small white flecks around perimeter of the iris
   _____ Most prominent on upper arms, shoulders, back
   _____ From pressure over occipitoparietal region during prolonged delivery
   _____ Telangiectatic nevi
   _____ Bluish-purple color of the hands and feet
   _____ Deep-blue pigmentation over lumbar and sacral areas

   A. Lanugo

   B. Cephalhematoma

   C. Acrocyanosis

   D. Mongolian spots

   E. Stork bites

   F. Cradle cap

   G. Harlequin color change

   H. Craniosynostosis

   I. Caput succedaneum

   J. Brushfield's spots

3. According to the rule of thumb for determining normal blood pressure values, what would be the expected normal blood pressure for a two-year-old child?

   _____
   _____
   _____
   _____
   _____

4. What are the *Apgar scores* for each of the following newborn caucasian infants?

	Infant A	Infant B	Infant C	Infant D
Heart rate	102	140	90	126
Respiratory rate	Slow, irregular	Crying vigorously	Slow, irregular	Crying
Muscle tone	Extremities slightly flexed	Active movement	Flaccid	Slight flexion
Reflex irritability	Grimaces	Crying	No response	Crying
Color	Body pink, extremities blue	Body pink, hands and feet blue	Cyanotic	Body pink, extremities blue
Apgar Score				

5. "When will my baby . . . "

   A. Cry real tears? _____
   B. Shiver when she's cold? _____
   C. Double his birth weight? _____
   D. Get her first tooth? _____
   E. Start his DTP shots? _____
   F. Really smile at me? _____

6. **True or False?**

☐ **T** ☐ **F**   Rooting and sucking reflexes are gone by the age of ten months.

☐ **T** ☐ **F**   Palpable pulsation in the anterior fontanel is normal.

☐ **T** ☐ **F**   The Babinski reflex usually disappears at the age of two years.

☐ **T** ☐ **F**   Chest circumference is greater than head circumference at one year.

☐ **T** ☐ **F**   Infants lose up to 10% of their birth weight by three days of age.

☐ **T** ☐ **F**   Fifty percent of all children develop an innocent murmur.

☐ **T** ☐ **F**   Visual acuity of the newborn is 20/100.

☐ **T** ☐ **F**   Tonsils graded 2+ at the age of ten are normal.

☐ **T** ☐ **F**   Genu varum (bow leg) is common from age two to four years.

☐ **T** ☐ **F**   Bronchovesicular breath sounds in the peripheral lung fields at the age of five are normal.

Lab Practice for The Complete Health and Physical Assessment

Chapter 24

Learning Objectives

1. Describe general documentation guidelines.
2. Identify characteristics of a successful assessment.
3. Demonstrate an integrated physical assessment on your lab partner.
4. Identify common documentation errors.

Reading Assignment

Prior to beginning this lab assignment, please read Chapter 24, "The Complete Health and Physical Assessment," in *Health Assessment & Physical Examination* by Mary Ellen Zator Estes, pages 773-793.

Laboratory Activities

1. What are some general documentation guidelines for clear and accurate written communication?

   _____
   _____
   _____
   _____
   _____

2. How should an error be corrected in documentation?

   _____
   _____
   _____
   _____
   _____

3. What is wrong with each of the following charted statements?

   A. *Patient states I have a really sore throat and a dry cough.*

   _____
   _____
   _____

B. *Patient catheterized for 550cc clear yellow urine. MS, RN*

_____

_____

_____

C. *Walking in hall occasionally with assistance.*

_____

_____

_____

D. *Patient appears to be having a good day today.*

_____

_____

_____

E. *Large abrasion noted on right arm.*

_____

_____

_____

F. *n/ cap refill*

_____

_____

_____

4. How can you obtain information for the mental status assessment?

_____

_____

_____

_____

5. What items in the health assessment are continuously evaluated?

_____

_____

_____

_____

6. How do you incorporate examination of the skin into your health assessment?

_____

_____

_____

_____

7. **Physical Exam.** *(Equipment: All items listed in previous chapters.)* Complete the *health history* and *review of systems* as noted in the text. Then, using your lab partner as a patient, follow the physical assessment guidelines (beginning on p. 776 in your text) to conduct an *integrated* physical assessment.

General Appearance _____

Neurological System _____

Measurements _____

Skin _____

Head and Face _____

Eyes _____

Ears _____

Nose and Sinuses _____

Mouth and Throat _____

Neck _____

Upper Extremities _____

Back, Posterior and Lateral Thoraxes _____

Anterior Thorax _____

Heart _____

Female Breasts _____

Male Breasts _____

Jugular Veins _____

Female and Male Breasts _____

Heart _____

Abdomen _____

Inguinal Area _____

Lower Extremities _____

Neurological System _____

Musculoskeletal System _____

Neurological System _____

Female Genitalia, Anus, Rectum _____

Male Genitalia _____

Male Anus, Rectum, Prostate _____

8. If you are examining an elderly patient, what steps can you take to make him more comfortable?

_____
_____
_____
_____
_____

What adjustments might you make in your assessment?

_____
_____
_____
_____
_____

9. How would you proceed with a patient who:

A. Seems hesitant about a having a particular part of the assessment performed?

_____
_____
_____
_____
_____

B. Refuses to answer certain questions?

_____
_____
_____
_____
_____

10. What reflexes would be assessed in the comatose patient?

_____
_____
_____
_____
_____

11. How can you show sensitivity when communicating bad news to a patient?

_____

_____

_____

_____

_____

Self-Assessment Quiz

1. True or False?

☐ T ☐ F   Correct another person's entry only if you know the information is false.

☐ T ☐ F   Incorporate assessment of any assistive devices into the physical examination.

☐ T ☐ F   Mental status is assessed prior to having the patient undress.

☐ T ☐ F   If possible, avoid abbreviations when documenting patient information.

☐ T ☐ F   Document any phone calls that relate to the patient's case.

☐ T ☐ F   Describe what you observed, not what you did.

☐ T ☐ F   Allow time after the physical exam to teach the patient self-assessment techniques.

2. How would you note an error in the following entry on a patient chart? (This patient was actually given a different medication.)

Pt. was medicated with Tylenol 650mg po at 1100 for pain in right lower leg.

3. Put the following assessments in the correct sequence for an integrated head-to-toe exam.

   A. Deep tendon reflexes

   B. Posterior thorax

   C. Anterior thorax

   D. Jugular veins

   E. Abdomen

   F. Genitalia

   G. Breasts

   H. Neck

   I. Ears

4. Let's translate: What do people *really* want to say when they use the following terms?

Ear drum _____

Adam's apple_____

Hammer (bone in middle ear)_____

Black and blue marks _____

Shoulder blades _____

Swollen glands _____

Womb _____

Breastbone _____

Ear wax _____

Soft spot _____

Knee cap _____

Taste buds _____

5. Your entire plan of care for a patient is based on _____.

Answers to Self-Assessment Quizzes

Chapter 1: The Nursing Process

1. Assessment, Nursing diagnosis, Planning, Implementation, Evaluation

2. | | |
    |---|---|
    | E | A, N |
    | P, I | P |
    | A | I |
    | P | E |
    | N | N |

3. | | |
    |---|---|
    | False | True |
    | True | True |
    | False | True |
    | False | |

4. B and D

5. Nursing care plan

Chapter 2: The Patient Interview

1. Active listening

2. Leading questions, Interrupting the patient, Talkativeness, Multiple questions, Using medical jargon

3. | | |
    |---|---|
    | False | True |
    | True | False |
    | True | False |

4. Exploring, Reflecting, Focusing, Encouraging comparisons, Normalizing

5. Defining appropriate boundaries, sharing personal reactions, refocusing the patient

Chapter 3: The Complete Health History

1. Complete, Episodic, Interval or follow-up, Emergency

2. E, G, G, I, A, B, D, F, C, G, I

3. False   False
    True   True
    True   False
    False

4. Not mentioned by the patient: Radiation, Quantity, Associated manifestations

5.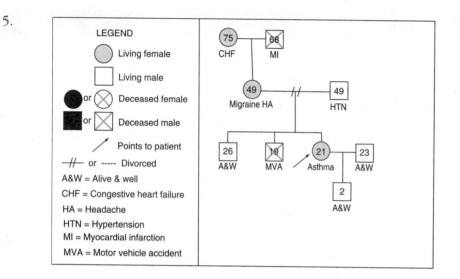

Chapter 4: Developmental Assessment

1. Erikson's epigenetic theory of personality

2. Young adult   Toddler
    Late middle adulthood   School-age children
    Preschooler   Adolescence
    Infancy

3. False   True
    True   True
    False   False

4. D, F, E, C, A, B

5. Life review

Chapter 5: Cultural Assessment

1. Culture

2. True   False
    False   True
    True   True
    False

3. 75% Euro-American
    12.3% African-American
    9% Hispanic
    2.8% Asian
    0.7% American Indian

4. Acculturation
    Culture shock

5. H, F, G, A, E, D, B, C

Chapter 6: Spiritual Assessment

1. Spiritual distress, Potential for enhanced spiritual well-being

2. False   False   False
    True   True   True
    False

3. A. Spirituality   C. Dogma   E. Spiritual distress
    B. Reincarnation   D. Animism

4. Platitude
    Cliché

5. A, H   H   I   B
    A   J, P   R   I
    A   J   I   R
    I, J, P, R, and sometimes B   B

Chapter 7: Nutritional Assessment

1. Health promotion
    Informs at-risk individuals of physical, cognitive, psychological, and social changes that occur
    Explains their nutritional needs

2. G, E, G and H, B, A, D, F, C, C, H, E

3. A. Fats, oils, and sweets.   B. Milk, yogurt, and cheese group.   C. Vegetable group.
    D. Meat, poultry, fish, dry beans, eggs, and nuts group.   E. Fruit group.   F. Bread, cereal,
    rice, and pasta group.

4. Patient C (due to probable insufficient calories and fluids for supporting breastfeeding)

5. A. 50–60%   B. 120%   C. 10-20%   D. 90%

6. "Do you have any concerns about your diet or eating?"

Chapter 8: Physical Assessment Techniques

1. Direct/immediate, Indirect/mediate, Direct fist, Indirect fist
    For the kidney—Fist percussion

2. False   True   False
    False   False
    True   True

3. A. Dorsal recumbent, B. Lithotomy, C. Sims', D. Semi-Fowler's

4. E, D, A, C, B, A, C

5. Validation of complaints   Monitor current health problems
    Screening of general well-being   Formulate diagnoses and treatments

Chapter 9: General Assessment and Vital Signs

1. G, I   C
    D, I, J   F
    J   H
    B   J
    D   H
    C

2. A. Temporal   D. Brachial   G. Popliteal
    B. Carotid   E. Radial   H. Posterior tibial
    C. Apical   F. Femoral   I. Dorsalis pedis

3. Ineffective pumping, Decreased circulating volume, Changes in characteristics of blood vessels, Diurnal variation

4. True   False
    False   True
    False   True
    True   False
    True

5. Circadian rhythm patterns, Hormones, Age, Exercise, Stress, Environmental extremes of hot and cold

Chapter 10: Skin, Hair, and Nails

1. Moisture, temperature, texture, turgor, edema, color, bleeding, ecchymosis, vascularity, lesions

2. C (180°)

3.   Tumor P   Papule P   Cyst P

      Keloid S   Fissure S   Lichenification S

      Erosion S   Ulcer S   Pustule P

      Vesicle P   Crust S   Scar S

4.   F, D, B, H, A, C, E, G

5.   Anterior chest, under the clavicle, abdomen

6.   A. Annular   C. Confluent

      B. Linear   D. Zosteriform

7.   A. Rubeola (measles)   B. Herpes zoster (shingles)

Chapter 11: Head and Neck

1.   Refer to your text, p. 267, Figure 11-3, Anterior and Posterior Cervical Triangles

2.   C, A, E, B, F, D

3.   A. Sternocleidomastoid muscle   F. Left lobe of thyroid

      B. Hyoid bone   G. Trachea

      C. Thyroid cartilage   H. Sternum

      D. Cricoid cartilage   I. Clavicle

      E. Isthmus of thyroid   J. Right lobe of thyroid

4.   Normal   Abnormal

      Abnormal   Abnormal

      Normal   Normal

Chapter 12: Eyes, Ears, Nose, Mouth, and Throat

1.   Fovea centralis

2.   F, G, I, B, H, J, D, A, C, E

3.   Pearly gray with clearly defined landmarks; distinct cone-shaped light reflex extending from the umbo at 5:00 position in the right ear and 7:00 position in the left; no bulging or retracting, no fluid, no perforations

4.   Lateralization to the left ear
      Bone conduction equal to or greater than air conduction in left ear

5.   Normal   Normal   Abnormal
      Abnormal   Normal   Normal

6.   Oral hairy leukoplakia, Mandibular tori, Scrotal tongue, Torus palatinus

Chapter 13: Breasts and Regional Nodes

1.   Location, size, shape, number, consistency, definition, mobility, tenderness, erythema, dimpling or retraction

2.   A, C, F, G

3.   Having a male patient lean forward is usually not necessary (except with gynecomastia)

4.   All are risk factors

5.   True   True
     False   False
     True   False

6.   A. Inspection: hands pressed against hips
     B. Palpation of supraclavicular nodes
     C. Palpation of infraclavicular nodes
     D. Bimanual palpation
     E. Palpation of axillary nodes
     F. Palpation of glandular tissue
     G. Palpation of the areola
     H. Compression of the nipple

Chapter 14: Thorax and Lungs

1.   A. Vesicular
     B. Increased carbon dioxide level, decreased oxygen level, increased blood pH level
     C. Long-standing hypoxia
     D. Crepitus

2.   E, G, F, B, D, C, A

3.   A. Tachypnea, B. Cheyne-Stokes, C. Kussmaul's, D. Biot's

4.   Patient A: Normal   Patient D: Abnormal
     Patient B: Abnormal   Patient E: Normal
     Patient C: Normal

5.   C   A   A, D
     B, D   A   A
     B, D   C

Chapter 15: Heart and Peripheral Vasculature

1.   Superior/inferior vena cava → right atrium → tricuspid valve → right ventricle → pulmonic valve → (pulmonary artery, lungs, pulmonary vein) → left atrium → mitral valve → left ventricle → aortic valve → aorta

2.
False	True
True	False
True	False
False	True
False	True

3. Refer to your text, p. 412, Figure 15-4 Events of the Cardiac Cycle

4. C, E, F, B, D, A

5. <u>Age</u>, <u>gender</u>, <u>race</u>, <u>family hx</u>, hypertension, hyperlipidemia, use of tobacco, diabetes, sedentary lifestyle, diet, stress, obesity

6. D, G, F, B, A, C, E

Chapter 16: Abdomen

1. Diaphragm, Symphysis pubis

2.
A	C
C	All
B	D
A	C and D
A	C

3.
Bell	Bell
Diaphragm	Diaphragm
Bell	Bell
Diaphragm	Both

4.
Normal	Abnormal
Normal	Normal
Abnormal	Normal
Normal	Abnormal
Abnormal	Abnormal

5. Fat, Fluid (ascites), Flatus, Feces, Fetus, Fatal growth (malignancy), Fibroid tumor

6.
A. Referred pain	E. Signs of discomfort or pain
B. Last	F. Gallbladder
C. Cough	G. Pain
D. Involuntary muscle guarding	H. Appendicitis

Chapter 17: Musculoskeletal System

1. C, G, H, F, D, E, A and B, B

2. 4 on a scale of 5

3.   False   True
        False   True
        False   False

4.   G, C, F, A, H, E, B, D

5.   All are true.

6.   A. Scoliosis, B. Lordosis, C. List, D. Kyphosis

7.   What is *straight leg raising test* (Lasègue's Test) or Milgram test

Chapter 18: Mental Status and Neurological Techniques

1.   G   H
        C   D
        B   A
        E

2.   Brachioradialis, Achilles, Patellar

3.   False   False
        True   True
        True   False
        True

4.   XI, IX and X, VII, II

5.   Nuchal rigidity, Kernig's sign, or Brudzinski's sign

Chapter 19: Female Genitalia

1.   Endocervical smear, Cervical smear, Vaginal pool smear

2.   False   True
        False   False
        True   True
        False   False

3.   A. Second
        B. Fourth
        C. Third
        D. First

4.   Trichomonas
        Candida

Venereal warts (Human papillomavirus—HPV)

Genital herpes (Herpes simplex)

5.   Positive Chandelier's sign

Chapter 20: Male Genitalia

1.   Hard, fixed area or nodules are palpated on the testicle.

2.   E, D, F, G, C, A, B

3.   The presence of bowel sounds

4.   False   False

      False   True

      True   False

      True

5.   Bloody or purulent penile discharge, Scrotal and/or testicular pain, Burning and/or pain on urination, Penile lesion

Chapter 21: Anus, Rectum, and Prostate

1.   Males over age 55, Having a first-degree relative with prostate cancer, African-American, High levels of serum testosterone

2.   G, D, E, A, F, C, B

3.   False   True

      True   False

      True   True

4.   Age over 55 years

5.   A. Thoracic expansion   D. Rectovaginal exam

      B. Palpation of spleen   E. Hepatojugular reflux

      C. Palpation of bulbourethral gland   F. Assessment of triceps reflex

Chapter 22: Pregnant Patient

1.   HCT 34%, Glucose screen

2.   A. 18-20 weeks   D. Which fetal part presents at the fundus

      B. 28 weeks   E. G: 1   P: 0

      C. 12 weeks   F. PIH

3.   D, E, H, I, B, C, A, G, F

4.   Leopold's maneuver
      A. Second
      B. First
      C. Fourth
      D. Third

5.   Normal   Normal
      Abnormal   Abnormal
      Normal   Normal

Chapter 23: Pediatric Patient

1.   16 pounds, 26 inches
      24 pounds, 29 inches

2.   G, H, F, B, J, A, I, E, C, D

3.   84/56

4.   6, 9, 2, 8

5.   A. 2-3 months   D. 5-7 months
      B. 6 months   E. 2 months
      C. 6 months   F. 2 months

6.   True   True
      True   False
      False   True
      False   False
      True   True

Chapter 24: The Complete Health and Physical Assessment

1.   False   True
      True   True
      True   False
      False

2.   *error 6/15/98 1130 Mary Smith, RN-* Pt. was medicated with Motrin

      Pt. was medicated with ~~Tylenol 650mg po~~ at 1100 for pain in right lower leg.   400 mg po at 1100 for pain in right lower leg.
      — 6115/98 1105 Mark Ramon, R.N.

3.   I. Ears   D. Jugular veins
      H. Neck   E. Abdomen
      B. Posterior thorax A. Deep tendon reflexes
      C. Anterior thorax   F. Genitalia
      G. Breasts

4. Tympanic membrane   Uterus

   Thyroid cartilage   Sternum

   Malleus   Cerumen

   Ecchymosis   (Anterior) fontanel

   Scapulae   Patella

   Lymphadenopathy (enlarged lymph nodes)   Papillae

5. Patient assessment